HIP REPLACEMENT

A PATIENT'S GUIDE TO SURGERY AND RECOVERY

Richard N. Villar,

MB BS BSc (Hons) MS FRCS

Consultant Orthopaedic Surgeon, Addenbrooke's Hospital,
Cambridge, United Kingdom
and
Clinical Director, Cambridge Hip and Knee Unit,
BUPA Cambridge Lea Hospital, Cambridge, United Kingdom

Thorsons
An Imprint of HarperCollinsPublishers

To Louise, Ruairidh, Angus and Felicity

Thorsons
An Imprint of HarperCollins*Publishers*
77–85 Fulham Palace Road,
Hammersmith, London W6 8JB
1160 Battery Street,
San Francisco, California 94111–1213

Published by Thorsons 1995
3 5 7 9 10 8 6 4 2 1

Text illustrations by Angela Christie

A catalogue record for this book is
available from the British Library

ISBN 0 7225 3169 9

Printed in Great Britain by
HarperCollinsManufacturing Glasgow

CONTENTS

ACKNOWLEDGEMENTS

It is impossible to do credit to all those who have helped me in the preparation of this book. I am bound to forget someone, so please forgive me if that someone happens to be you.

Specific thanks must go to my colleagues and staff at Addenbrooke's Hospital, Cambridge, and the Cambridge Hip and Knee Unit at the BUPA Cambridge Lea Hospital. My thanks also to those who perused the various chapters and gave excellent advice: John Collis, Nancy Jordan, and the Department of Physiotherapy at Addenbrooke's Hospital, Cambridge. And what would I do without my secretaries who are able to convert my garbled dictation into reasonable prose? Eternal thanks to the 'boss', Jenny Kenworthy, and her team of Linda Phillips and Hazel Byrne. Finally, I owe much to Jane Graham-Maw of Thorsons who kept me working very much to time, and ensured that my family holiday was largely spent at a portable wordprocessor. But my biggest thank you must go to my patients – past and present – without whom I would never have been in the position to write a book such as this. *You* have been my biggest stimulus. You are truly wonderful, the lot of you.

1

INTRODUCTION

Hip replacement has revolutionized the lives of many patients. Worldwide, more than 500 000 are undertaken each year. Large though this number may be, it continues to increase.

Frequently called *total* hip replacement (THR) or *total hip arthroplasty* (THA), the operation has now become available to a wide spectrum of patients. Such patients are often of quite a young age. When initially introduced as a new procedure, it was widely recommended that the operation should not be performed on patients under the age of 65, but, now, younger individuals receive a hip replacement, frequently with out-standing success. The transformation of the individual's life from one of crippling pain to one of mobile happiness is now widely accepted.

A patient awaiting hip replacement will frequently experience a dramatic decline in quality of life. Pain can be very debilitating and dominate every aspect of daily living. Sleep at night can be disturbed, tempers can be lost easily during trivial family disagreements and time away from work can put employment in peril. With a successful hip replacement, though, all of this can be reversed. As a surgeon, I have noticed that the patient benefits because the pain disappears, but that the whole family feels better too as a result.

Patient satisfaction following hip replacement is greater than for any other operation available worldwide today. Though coronary bypasses compete hotly for first position, more than 95 per cent of patients say that they are extremely happy with their hip replacement after it has been performed. It is hip replacement, more than any other operation, that has made orthopaedic surgery such a high-demand specialty.

There are many reasons for performing a hip replacement operation. Perhaps the commonest is osteoarthritis, otherwise known as degenerative disease of the hip joint. As people live longer, and as other surgical advances improve the quality of life, so more people require hip replacement. In certain countries of the world, long waiting lists exist for orthopaedic surgery. From time to time, government pressure will create a waiting list initiative, with large numbers of hip replacements being performed in a short space of time. All of these factors contribute to the increasing numbers of hip replacements being performed.

Though hip replacement is a major operation, the chances of its resulting in complications are relatively low. Being of man-made material, some hip replacements will fail if left in place for long enough. None the less, the ten-year survival time of most designs is excellent and the improvement they make to the quality of life during that time is remarkable.

Though survival rates of hip replacements in excess of 20 years are now regularly being reported, it is safer to say that the average hip replacement will usually last 10 years.

Once it does fail, it is theoretically possible to perform another replacement. This is referred to as a *revision* procedure. Revision surgery is more complicated than the initial replacement (often referred to as the *primary* replacement). Indeed, in the recent past, the revision operation was considered to be a substandard operation, the only real hope any patient had of a successful hip replacement being the first time round. However, as increasing numbers of primary hip replacements have been performed, the subspecialty of revision hip surgery has appeared. This has become associated with specialist instrumentation, detailed pre-operative investigations and the facility of banking bone for transplantation. As a consequence, in some hospitals, revision hip replacement can now vie keenly with primary hip replacement as regards long-term survival. Revisions of revisions can now be performed, and such revisions can also be further revised. It is perhaps fair to say, though, that, despite such improvements in technique, a revision hip replacement may not perform as well as a primary hip replacement and is best avoided if possible.

Despite the popularity and success of hip replacement, patients are often given little pre-operative information about it. This is despite the obvious ethical right to know what to expect. Anyone should be able to ask the kinds of questions that will inform them about the procedure. Why does a hip replacement need to be performed at all? If it does need to be performed, should any one, specific technique be used? What are the chances of complications? How long will it last? The list of questions is endless, but the information generally available sparse. Many texts on the subject exist for surgeons and paramedical staff, but patients are frequently confined to obtaining what little information they can from hospital pamphlets, brief consultations with operation staff and the like. It is the purpose of this book to reverse this situation.

Within these pages can be found a general overview of the subject of hip replacement. It should be remembered that not *all* hip replacements are performed in the same way, nor do they all behave similarly after surgery. The nature of a book such as this is that it is necessary to generalize when, in reality, each person's precise situation has to be taken into account. However, what this book can do is give you a sound knowledge of hip replacement as an operation and an understanding of what can be regarded as a normal result, or, for that matter, an abnormal one. Remember that arthritis of the hip is not a new disease, even prehistoric man suffered from it (see Figure 1.1), but could not have a hip replacement operation. Remember also that everything I say in these pages is my own opinion. So if you have any doubts at all — ask your surgeon!

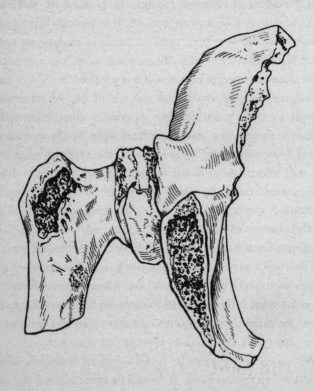

Figure 1.1 *Osteoarthritis of the hip. Note the irregular joint surface and osteophyte formation. This hip joint was excavated from an old Anglo-Saxon burial ground. Even ancient man was not spared the agony of arthritis.*

2

ANATOMY

This chapter will undoubtedly be the hardest to understand and read, but is very useful as it is an overview of the language used by medical staff when discussing and describing the various parts of the body. If you have no idea what the medical terms used mean, it makes things that much harder to take in. I have tried to explain this complicated subject as simply as possible, but if you still find it unreadable and indigestible, then simply look at the pictures and read on. Come back to it later and you will probably find it easier to understand.

Anatomy is a difficult subject and one that takes up quite a lot of time in a doctor's training. This is because it is vital to fully understand how the body works. To consider the anatomy of the hip joint is not only to consider the bones involved, but the muscles, nerves, blood vessels and many other structures that make up the whole.

The Hip Joint

The hip joint is the largest joint in the body and is referred to as a *ball-and-socket* joint. The ball is created by the spherical upper end of the thigh bone (*femur*), while the socket (*acetabulum*) is on the outer side of the pelvic bone.

In order that a joint may create limited friction when it moves, the bony surfaces that form the joints are covered with gristle (*articular cartilage*). This gristle, combined with a small amount of greasy fluid – called *synovial fluid* – allows the joint to function smoothly and painlessly for many years.

The hip joint is a weight-bearing joint, taking the full force of the weight of the upper body when you walk. The same could not be said, for example, of the shoulder joint.

DEVELOPMENT

The first signs of a hip joint developing can be seen in the embryo after only eight weeks. Bones do not initially appear in their bony form at all, but start off as cartilage and gradually change into bone.

The acetabulum in the embryo and young child consists of three different bones, the:

- *ilium*
- *ischium*
- *pubis.*

As development proceeds, so these cartilaginous structures become ossified (turn into bone) and fuse with one another to form the acetabulum and pelvis.

By the time you are between 15 and 25, the hip joint has developed and growth in that area ceases. Growth in the human body does not stop simultaneously in all parts of the skeleton, but ceases in a staggered manner over many years.

FEMUR

The femur (see Figure 2.1) is a very long bone, strong and very thick. At its upper end is the hip joint and at its lower end is the knee joint. Its long, straight portion, the *femoral shaft*, is not truly straight, but slightly bowed in a forwards direction. In anatomical parlance, the word 'forwards' is *anterior*, while 'backwards' is *posterior*, and 'upwards' is *superior* and 'downwards' is *inferior*. Thus, the femoral shaft is bowed *anteriorly*. Again, speaking anatomically, the lower end of the bone is the *distal* end, while the upper end is the *proximal* end. The knee joint is thus at the distal end of the femur and the hip joint at its proximal end.

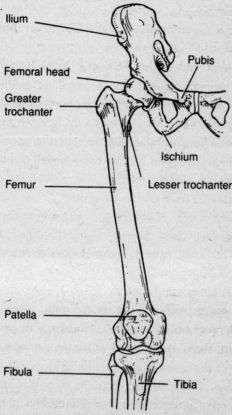

Ilium

Pubis

Femoral head

Greater trochanter

Ischium

Femur

Lesser trochanter

Patella

Fibula

Tibia

Figure 2.1 *The femur and pelvis.*

The ball at the proximal end of the femur is the *femoral head*. It is this ball that articulates with the acetabulum. The ball is connected to the *shaft* of the femur by means of the *femoral neck*. The femoral neck is attached to the shaft at an angle of approximately 140 degrees (the *neck/shaft angle*) and is also twisted slightly forwards, a phenomenon known as *anteversion*. If the neck was twisted in a backwards direction, this would be called *retroversion*. In hip replacement surgery, if the artificial hip is anteverted or retroverted too far when it is inserted during the operation, this can sometimes lead to post-operative dislocation. An understanding of the concepts of neck/shaft angles, anteversion, and retroversion, is therefore very important for the surgeon.

At the upper end of the shaft, and at the bottom of the neck, is a large lump of bone referred to as the *greater trochanter*. When most non-medical people are asked to point to their own hip joint, they point to the greater trochanter. This is the hard lump of bone that can be felt to one side at the top of the thigh, provided you are not too well padded there! In reality, though, the hip joint itself is a good 9 cm (3½ in) beyond this point, deep within the groin.

On the inner side of the femur, just below the femoral neck, is another bony bump, which is called the *lesser trochanter*. This is where certain muscles are attached.

ACETABULUM

The acetabulum is the socket of the hip joint. It is not actually a true socket, because its inferior margin is open. Like the femoral head, the socket is lined with articular cartilage, but, in the case of the acetabulum, this lining does not cover the whole surface. The articular cartilage layer is shaped like a horseshoe, open inferiorly, and is referred to as the *lunate* surface of the acetabulum.

In the centre of the horseshoe is a small cavity called the *cotyloid fossa* (the word 'fossa' is given to small pits and cavities that are found in various parts of the human body).

The deepest part of the acetabulum, the innermost part, is often referred to as the *medial wall*. The term 'medial' is an anatomical word used to describe a part of the body as being close to the *midline*. The midline is an imaginary vertical line joining the nose and belly button, which is extended to the ground when you stand. The term *lateral* is used when the part is further away from the midline. The greater trochanter, for example, is lateral to the femoral head. The medial wall of the acetabulum is therefore its deepest part and separates the acetabulum itself from all of the structures within the pelvic cavity. These structures include the ovaries and womb, bladder, bowels and many other soft tissue organs and structures.

THE SOFT TISSUES OF THE HIP

Those unfamiliar with human anatomy think that the hip joint consists entirely of bone and gristle, but, in fact, it consists of much more. There are soft tissues in the hip (see Figure 2.2) and they play a very important part in its overall function.

Between the femoral head and the acetabulum, running from the cotyloid fossa to a small pit in the middle of the femoral head (the *fovea*) is a ligament. This ligament is the *ligamentum teres* and it is very thick and strong. Its true function is unknown, but it can carry a large blood vessel in the developing hip.

The open inferior aspect of the acetabulum is also bridged by a ligament, the *transverse ligament*. With this ligament is usually found a wafer-like structure called the *labrum*, which surrounds the whole of the margin of the acetabulum. The labrum has a number of functions. Some surgeons believe it exists to deepen the acetabular socket still further, while

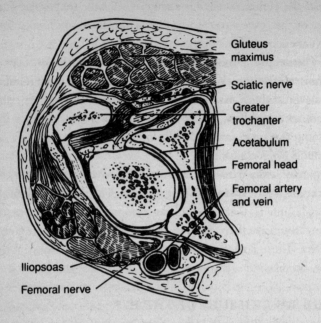

Gluteus maximus

Sciatic nerve

Greater trochanter

Acetabulum

Femoral head

Femoral artery and vein

Iliopsoas

Femoral nerve

Figure 2.2 *A cross-section of the hip joint showing the major anatomical structures.*

others believe that the labrum acts like a buffer, in the same way that a cartilage does within the knee.

The whole of the hip joint is surrounded by a thick tissue envelope called the *capsule*. This is a strong structure, reinforced at a number of points by ligaments. The capsule attaches to the margin of the acetabulum at its superior end and to the neck of the femur at its inferior end. Because it is attached quite some way down the femoral neck, it is possible for an infection within the shaft of the upper femur to burst through the bone and extend into the hip joint.

The inner aspect of the capsule is lined by a thin membrane called the *synovium*. Sometimes referred to as the *synovial membrane*, it is this which is partly responsible for the production of the greasy *synovial fluid* that lubricates and nourishes the articular surfaces of the joint. The healthy hip joint moves very smoothly – more smoothly than a skate on ice – with almost no friction. When the joint surfaces become irregular, however, which happens in many hip diseases, friction becomes a problem.

BLOOD VESSELS
Blood vessels are to be found both within the hip joint and immediately around it. Over the front of the hip joint (anteriorly) lies the *femoral artery*. This is the main artery taking blood from the upper body to the leg. Two *gluteal* arteries may also be found in the vicinity of the hip, the *superior gluteal* and the *inferior gluteal*.

As well as these main arteries, the area of the hip joint is rich in blood supply and there are many other smaller vessels that contribute to its function and health. Alongside every artery its corresponding vein is to be found. The arteries are the blood vessels that carry blood away from the heart, the blood then being full of oxygen. The veins carry blood back to the heart after the tissues have been supplied with the oxygen they need.

NERVES
Three nerves may be found within the vicinity of the hip joint, the:

* *femoral nerve*
* *sciatic nerve*
* *obturator nerve*.

The femoral nerve is immediately adjacent to the femoral

artery anterior to the hip joint. The sciatic nerve is situated immediately behind the hip joint. The obturator nerve is quite some distance from the hip joint itself, being quite medially situated, but it does help provide the nerve supply to the soft tissues around the joint. For the surgeon, the nerves that cause concern are the sciatic and the femoral nerves. Depending on the surgical approach used, both can be damaged during surgery. Great care is taken together with attention to detail to ensure that this risk is minimized.

MUSCLES

Without muscles, the hip joint would not be able to move. The muscles that surround the joint are extremely powerful, but, then, if these major muscles do not work at full strength, it is very difficult for a patient to walk without a limp.

The most important muscles around the hip are the *gluteal* muscles as these support the joint. There are three muscles that make up this group, the:

- *gluteus maximus*
- *gluteus medius*
- *gluteus minimus.*

Birth defects of the hip joint or longstanding hip disease can cause the gluteal muscles to become ineffective. This can also be the result of paralytic conditions, such as polio. When this happens, the patient walks with what is called a *dipping gait*. Surgeons sometimes refer to this as a *positive Trendelenburg gait*, named after the famous surgeon who originally described a test for gluteal muscle weakness.

The gluteal muscles make up the buttocks and, thus, are largely to be found on the lateral and posterior aspects of the hip joint. A longer, thinner muscle called the *tensor fascia lata* may also be found on the lateral aspect of the hip and thigh.

On the inner thigh, though a fair distance away from the hip joint, may be found another broad muscle mass, called the *adductor* muscles. Though these are not closely linked with the functioning of the hip joint itself, they do materially influence its movement. What they do exactly is described later.

Over the front of the hip joint may be found a very tough muscle called the *psoas*. It starts from within the abdomen, attaching to some of the vertebrae, passes over the front of the hip joint and inserts into the lesser trochanter.

Two other muscles found on the front of the hip joint, separating the hip joint from the femoral artery and nerve, are the *pectineus* and *iliacus*. The iliacus and psoas muscles lie very close together over the front of the hip joint. The combination of the two is referred to as the *iliopsoas*.

Close by is another powerful muscle, the *rectus femoris*. It is attached proximally from the pelvis.

Lying over the posterior side of the hip joint are a number of smaller muscles, frequently with long, complicated names.

MOVEMENTS

For a hip joint to function normally, it must be able to travel through its full range of movement. Surgeons break down the various movements of the hip into their component parts. Bending of the joint is referred to as *flexion*, while straightening is *extension*. Twisting the joint inwards is *internal rotation*, while twisting outwards is *external rotation*. Lifting the leg sideways is referred to as *abduction*, while crossing one leg over the other is *adduction*.

With longstanding hip disease, it is possible for some, or all, of these movements to become impossible. If that happens, then a *fixed deformity* is said to occur and then certain muscles that surround the hip joint can begin to shorten.

Once they do, it is called a *contracture*.

The commonest contracture of the hip joint is the flexion contracture — when the hip joint slowly flexes and will no longer straighten. This can also happen after hip surgery. A significant part of a physiotherapist's efforts are thus aimed at reducing the chances of flexion contracture occurring after the operation.

Hip movements cannot be considered in isolation. The actions of the hip also influence other joints in the body, though predominantly the knee and the spine. When a hip joint begins to lose its normal range of movement, extra strain can be placed on both spine and knee. It is not uncommon for patients with severe loss of hip movement, for whatever reason, to also complain of back pain. Indeed, occasionally hips have been replaced in order to relieve pressure on the spine.

The different muscles surrounding the hip joint are responsible for different movements. Gluteal muscles, for example, lying largely on the lateral and posterior aspects of the joint, are responsible for either abduction or extension. The muscles on the front of the hip joint are responsible for hip flexion, though the psoas also causes internal rotation. The adductor muscles, lying on the inner side of the thigh, cause hip joint adduction.

3

THE HISTORY AND DEVELOPMENT OF HIP REPLACEMENT SURGERY

For generations, surgeons have been faced with the problem of how to treat the painful hip. Replacement is only one of many different treatment options available and so it is worth considering the alternatives at this stage, as this will give a better idea of why it has become so successful. It should also be remembered that even today, in the 1990s, many of the alternatives are still used in special situations. For example, a patient may be so young that hip replacement seems ill-advised or a surgeon may be practising in a less developed part of the world without the necessary facilities for the operation.

The alternatives, which form part of the development of hip replacement, that will be considered here are as follows:

- injection
- forage, cheilectomy and joint clearance
- denervation
- muscle release
- excision arthroplasty
- arthrodesis
- osteotomy
- arthroscopy

Let us now look at each of these in turn.

Injection

Though it could be argued that an injection is not truly a surgical procedure, it does represent an important part of the early management of a painful hip joint.

It involves the introduction, by a needle, of a combination of local anaesthetic and steroid into the joint. Sometimes this injection is given while observing the joint by means of X-ray. Because the hip joint is located deep inside the body, this measure ensures that the needle is accurately located to deliver the drugs.

The steroid comes in a variety of forms, the commonest used in such a situation being hydrocortisone acetate. A longer-acting version is triamcinolone. Both of these substances exert an anti-inflammatory effect on the hip joint and can help with pain relief as a result. Repeated injections into a joint, however, can eventually cause damage in themselves and so many practitioners will not undertake more than a limited number for any one patient for this reason.

The effect of such an injection can sometimes be miraculous, though the more severely damaged a hip joint is, the less likely it is that the injection will have a satisfactory effect.

The length of time for which an injection may provide pain relief is also variable, but periods of six months or longer are not unusual. An injection does not always have an instantaneous effect and it may take as long as two or three weeks before any benefit is experienced.

Forage, Cheilectomy and Joint Clearance

Forage is a rarely used surgical procedure that attempts to increase the blood supply within the bone surrounding a joint. It involves making multiple drill holes and saw cuts in the hip joint area on the basis that once a damaged area has been stimulated, it has the opportunity to recover.

Cheilectomy involves the removal of damaged articular cartilage in the hope that this will either regrow or be replaced by less painful tissue.

Joint clearance is an operation whereby the hip joint is opened and cleared of loose particulate matter, with irregular surfaces being trimmed down.

None of these three operations has been outstandingly successful. In most cases, they have either failed or only produced limited relief. However, until the late 1960s, such procedures were being widely practised as, in certain hands, encouraging results were said to have been obtained. By 1967, though, it became apparent that these options should largely be abandoned because results were not sufficiently reliable.

Denervation

Pain is felt as a result of impulses transmitted along nerves. Denervation may be performed either surgically or by injection. Performing denervation surgically involves the division of a branch of the obturator nerve. Results are unpredictable, with success only being achieved in 50 per cent of cases and then only for a limited period.

Performing denervation by injection involves introducing local anaesthetic to the area where the nerves surrounding the hip joint (femoral, sciatic and obturator) are located. Local anaesthetic only lasts for a limited period of time, but it has been noticed that the pain-relieving effects of such an injection can last for a significant period after the local anaesthetic itself should have disappeared. Quite why this should be the case is difficult to say, but, for a patient who is otherwise unable to be offered surgery, it can be a technique worth considering.

Muscle Release Operations

Nobody truly knows why an arthritic hip is painful. The detailed mechanisms that mean pain is felt in such a circumstance are not easily explained. One theory is that pain is felt because of an increase in pressure within the hip joint. This pressure is in part created by the high tension of the strong muscles that surround the joint. If these muscles are divided, then the tension is theoretically reduced. Muscle division (known as muscle *release*) has been proposed as a possible treatment. If a large number of hip muscles are divided, this procedure is sometimes referred to as the *hanging hip* operation.

Though no longer widely practised, such operations may form part of other procedures, rather than being used in isolation. They are of limited value by themselves.

Excision arthroplasty

Excision arthroplasty is an operation whereby the hip joint is surgically removed (*excised*). The removal of a structure is also referred to as resection. This operation is therefore sometimes called *resection arthroplasty*.

Excision arthroplasty was first described in 1928 as a treatment of choice for tuberculosis and infection of the hip joint.

It involved the resection of the femoral head and the rim of the acetabulum. Some of the gluteal muscles were also excized at the same time.

The operation was proposed by a Mr Gathorne Girdlestone (1881–1950) who practised in Oswestry and Oxford, United Kingdom, and was the first Professor of Orthopaedic Surgery in Great Britain. In 1945, Girdlestone proposed excision arthroplasty as a treatment for osteoarthritis of the hip joint, though there were a number of minor differences between the excision arthroplasty he proposed for osteoarthritis and that which he had proposed earlier for tuberculosis. The operation for osteoarthritis preserved the greater trochanter and was followed by an eight-week period in bed. Because of the work of Professor Girdlestone, excision arthroplasty is sometimes referred to as a *Girdlestone procedure*.

Surprisingly, patients are able to be mobile after an excision arthroplasty. An individual would not be described as nimble, but is able to move about. Approximately 50 per cent of patients will require crutches or two walking sticks to walk, but as many as 25 per cent can walk without any form of hand-held aid to enable them to do so.

Excision arthroplasty is now kept as an operation of last resort when a hip replacement has failed. If there is no hope of reconstructing a severely damaged hip replacement, then the Girdlestone operation is performed as what is called a *salvage procedure*.

Arthrodesis

Arthrodesis is a term that describes the surgical fusion of a joint, fused so that it is no longer capable of movement. The operation can be performed in a number of ways and was widely undertaken in the past following infections of the hip joint, particularly tuberculosis. It is a highly effective method of controlling pain in the hip, but at the expense of all movement.

Though successful in controlling pain, the operation is now rarely performed because of the effect it can have on surrounding joints. Once the hip is fused, more stress is placed on the knee and spine. It is therefore not unusual for patients to develop long-term back pain or long-term osteoarthritic changes within the knee. This can happen many years later, presenting the surgeon with a situation that is very difficult to treat.

Some claim that an arthrodesis can later be converted to a total hip replacement. In reality, this is quite a simple operation to perform, sometimes being recommended to protect a deteriorating knee or spine. However, when a joint has been fused for many years and the muscles around it have become weak and ineffective, hip replacement frequently gives an unsatisfactory result.

Even if a hip replacement is performed successfully following an arthrodesis, the patient frequently walks with a dipping gait thereafter because the muscles cannot regain full strength and activity after such a lengthy period of fusion. Despite these disadvantages, arthrodesis is still a realistic option in certain cases of osteoarthritis.

Osteotomy

The word osteotomy is used to describes the division of a bone. The surgeon will often perform an osteotomy using either a saw or an instrument called an *osteotome*. This is a surgical chisel, though the shape of the tip is slightly different to the chisel that many of us would use at home.

An osteotomy is performed as a means of altering the way

that the strain of the weight of the body is passed through the hip joint. When you walk, stresses pass up the shaft of the femur, along the femoral neck, through the femoral head and thence into the hip joint. If an osteotomy is performed through the femur just above the level of the lesser trochanter, the angle of the femoral neck (the neck/shaft angle – see page 8) can be altered. This, in turn, ensures that the forces of walking pass through the femoral head in a different way. Areas of undiseased articular cartilage that were not initially involved in cushioning the joint can now be brought into play, potentially allowing diseased areas to heal.

Osteotomies are still widely performed, though not as frequently as hip replacement operations. Surgeons who undertake an osteotomy do so because they believe that the procedure may serve the purpose of being a useful holding operation before hip replacement is undertaken. Though the results of an osteotomy are difficult to predict, patients who have a reasonable range of movement in the hip before surgery and for whom osteoarthritis is only mild to moderate tend to do better than those with severe disease. As a rough guide, it can be said that 70 to 80 per cent of patients will feel benefit for 1 to 2 years after having had an osteotomy, but after 5 years this percentage will be 50 per cent and by 10 years it will be approximately 30 per cent.

None the less, osteotomy is a realistic surgical choice in some cases. This is particularly so for younger people. However, it should not be compared with hip replacement. The purpose of the osteotomy is to try and delay the need for hip replacement, not to act as a substitute for it. It is a major operation in its own right and carries with it the chances of certain complications. However, once the osteotomy has failed, however many years after surgery that may be, the patient is then in a position to receive a total hip replacement.

The risks of hip replacement are slightly greater following an osteotomy than if the osteotomy had never been performed. This should also be borne in mind when the decision as to whether or not to perform an osteotomy is being made. It is highly recommended that all patients discuss the technical difficulties of the procedure, the likely long-term results and the effect on any subsequent hip replacement with their orthopaedic surgeon before making a final decision for or against it.

Arthroscopy

The arthroscopy operation involves passing a small viewing telescope into a joint — most often the knee and, more recently, the shoulder. Its use in the hip is relatively new.

In arthroscopy — otherwise known as *keyhole* orthopaedic surgery — a small viewing telescope is introduced into the hip joint and the surgeon operates through other small holes adjacent to the viewing hole. The telescope used is only 4.5 mm (³⁄₁₆ in) in diameter (the telescope used for children is only 2.7 mm (about ²⁄₁₆ in).

It allows good access to the hip joint and is an excellent way to assess the condition of the hip. It is useful, for example, in establishing whether or not an osteotomy is likely to be helpful. It is also a very good way of performing a joint clearance and is more convenient for the patient as they only need to stay in hospital for about 36 hours. Also stitches are rarely required as the incisions are tiny, healing themselves within five to six days without stitches.

The success of arthroscopy in the treatment of osteoarthritis is difficult to predict at the time of writing as clinical trials have only recently begun to be performed. However, for patients who are 55 or younger, with only mild to moderate osteoarthritis and for whom the range of movement within the hip is fair, 70 per cent are likely to experience pain relief for at least a couple of years – the remaining 30 per cent showing little benefit from the procedure. It is unlikely, however, that hip arthroscopy will make symptoms *worse* in the long term and, further, it does not interfere with the surgeon's ability to perform a hip replacement in the years to come.

Joint Replacement

It is because of the unpredictability of alternative methods of treatment that joint replacement (see Figure 3.1) has become the surgical procedure that is most widely used to treat the painful hip.

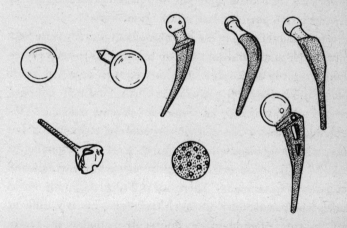

Figure 3.1 *A selection of hip replacement components. Top row (left to right): Interposition arthroplasty cup (Smith-Petersen), metal Judet prosthesis, banana stem femoral component, Charnley femoral component, modern straight stem modular component.*
Bottom row (left to right): Screw stem acetabular component (cementless), modern porous-coated acetabular component (cementless), straight stem cementless femoral component.

Though many are now performed, a hip replacement is not a new operation at all. The first was performed by a Dr Gluck in 1891 and all manner of types of hip replacement have developed since those days. In 1926, Professor Hey Groves (1872–1944) described the use of an ivory femoral head replacement to overcome painful osteoarthritis of the hip. This involved replacing the femoral head with half of an ivory sphere, attached to which was a long peg that passed down the femoral neck, emerging at the base of the greater trochanter.

At about this time, not only were various designs of hip replacement being considered, but the importance of maintaining sterile conditions during surgery was also being addressed. Orthopaedic surgery – and, in particular, the fixing of fractures and joint replacement – frequently involves implanting man-made materials into patients. As soon as this is undertaken, a natural risk of infection exists.

Operating theatres in the late nineteenth century were fairly primitive affairs and so it was up to surgeons to keep everything as sterile as possible. As a consequence, Sir Arbuthnot Lane (1857–1943), a surgeon at Guy's Hospital, London, originated what is now known as the *no-touch technique*. This technique ensures that neither surgeon nor assistant touches the patient's incision with their hands from the beginning to the end of the operation. The entire procedure is conducted with sterile instruments. There are still surgeons in the world today who practice the no-touch technique, but it is difficult and, in view of modern developments in operating theatre design, is probably no longer necessary.

As well as improvements in operative technique, the development of hip replacements continued. In 1936, Mr P. Wiles introduced a *total* hip replacement, where both the femoral head and the acetabulum were replaced with metal ones. This was referred to as a *metal-to-metal* total prosthesis. The components used were fixed to the bones with screws.

At about the same time, some surgeons began to feel that there was no point in replacing the whole hip when the disease process only affected a small part of it. For this reason, an operation referred to as *cup arthroplasty* or *interposition arthroplasty* was proposed by a Mr M. Smith-Petersen in 1939. This involved applying a metal cup over the damaged femoral head and this was then interposed between femoral head and acetabulum.

Such surface replacements did not do particularly well and, thus, in 1946, the Judet brothers in France proposed their own hip replacement. This was a very similar design to the ivory replacement of 30 years earlier, but it was made from acrylic. In the short term these did well, but they were not sufficiently strong to withstand the stresses and strains over an extended period of time and many fractured or became loose. The Judet replacement also had the annoying habit of squeaking loudly whenever the patient walked!

In the 1950s, some surgeons were still attempting to replace just the femoral head, despite the earlier work by Wiles with *total* hip replacements. A total hip replacement is exactly that – replacement of the *whole* hip joint, which is the acetabulum and femoral head. Replacement of the femoral head alone is sometimes referred to as *hemiarthroplasty*, which means the replacement of only half the hip joint. Austin Moore (1952) and F. Thompson (1954) both designed hemiarthroplasties for arthritis sufferers. However, it was soon established that these prostheses did not achieve fully satisfactory results in osteoarthritic patients, though they are still widely used when treating patients who have fractured a hip, even today.

At the same time that Moore and Thompson were proposing their hemiarthroplasties, work was being done to expand the possibilities of total hip replacement, in much the same way as Wiles had proposed in 1936.

In 1951, Kenneth McKee, a surgeon from Norwich, United Kingdom, proposed his metal-to-metal total prosthesis. This design worked very well for large numbers of patients.

However, in 1959, modern hip replacement can be said to have been born. In that year, John Charnley, from England, proposed the insertion of a hip replacement into a patient, but fixed it to the patient's bones with an acrylic cement. It was the arrival of this cement that dramatically improved how the hip replacement performed.

Charnley (1911–1982) subsequently became Sir John Charnley and continued to work exhaustively in the field of hip replacement surgery until his death. He introduced the concept of careful research and design prior to a component being used at surgery, and also recognized the importance of regular follow-up appointments with patients after their operations to check that all was as it should be. Only in this way could improvements be made. Even today, many decades after Sir John Charnley published the results of his first operation, the performance of modern hip replacements is still compared to the 'Charnley standard'. Though many orthopaedic surgeons have done much to advance the current standing of hip replacement, Sir John Charnley perhaps made the biggest single contribution to its development.

4

WHY REPLACE THE HIP?

When faced with an array of different surgical options that could be used for the hip joint, why replace the hip at all? The fact is that, for a wide variety of conditions, a hip replacement is the best option for treating them. The results can be better and last longer than those of other options, even when the problem of failure is taken into account. Nevertheless, it is always worth considering whether or not any other surgical options are applicable before deciding to undertake a hip replacement (see Chapter 3 for outlines of the alternatives).

The hip is replaced because of the symptoms a person experiences, not just because they have a particular condition. There are three main symptoms that would suggest that a hip replacement should be carried out:

- pain
- deformity
- the other joints are suffering because of the hip and need to be protected.

Pain

The overriding reason for performing a hip replacement operation is that of the need to control pain. The commonest cause
of pain in the hip is osteoarthritis, often referred to as *degenerative disease*, or 'wear and tear'. A hip replacement operation
is an excellent way to relieve such pain, but it is important that
both surgeon and patient consider pre-operatively whether
the pain level is sufficient to justify undertaking such a major
procedure. If replacement is performed when pain levels are
not high, the result can be disappointing for the patient.
However, if a patient has had unremitting, deep-seated pain
for many months or years, the effect of a total hip replacement
can be dramatic. The pain resulting from the degenerative disease disappears almost immediately after surgery – indeed,
patients frequently find that their pain has gone on waking up
after the operation. There is obviously the discomfort of the
surgery itself, but this settles within a few days.

When trials have been performed on total hip replacement,
researchers have found that it is possible to quantify the level
of discomfort the patient is feeling. If the levels of pain are
quantified both before and after surgery, a dramatic improvement is found. Pain is obviously very subjective and what is
intolerable for one patient may be acceptable to another. Also,
it is not always possible to relate the degree of discomfort a
patient feels to the severity of osteoarthritis they have.
Surgeons frequently see patients and their X-rays show that
they have chronic osteoarthritis, yet they seem to feel very little pain. Other patients' X-rays show no notable changes and
yet they experience unremitting, relentless discomfort.

The decision whether or not to undertake a total hip
replacement is thus primarily based on the clinical assessment

of the patient. X-rays and other investigations, certainly in the early stages, can confuse the issue. It is what the patient tells the surgeon that counts.

Classic hip pain can be felt in a number of areas around the hip joint. The commonest area is deep within the groin. For this reason, many cases of osteoarthritis of the hip are diagnosed as groin strains in the early stages, before X-rays show up abnormalities. Pain can also be felt over the greater trochanter, buttock and the thigh.

When considering pain, the concept of *referred* pain should be discussed. Though the majority of patients with arthritic hip joints feel pain within the hip, this is not always the case. Many can feel pain referred to the knee and sometimes even further down the leg. A recent study showed that 30 per cent of patients with osteoarthritis of the hip felt pain not only in the hip, but down to the knee and beyond.

Just as hip pain can be referred to areas other than the hip, pain in the hip can be referred from elsewhere. For example, pain from the spine can be referred to the hip area, as can pain from the soft tissues within the pelvis. An ovarian cyst or a hernia or even problems with the prostate gland in men can occasionally present as hip pain. These are unusual situations, but they should be borne in mind by any practitioner assessing a patient with a painful hip joint.

Because of the various locations in which hip pain may be felt, combined with the problem of referred pain, it is sometimes difficult to diagnose why patients are feeling discomfort and from where the discomfort originates. Tests do exist to help in making such a diagnosis, but there still remains a small group of patients for whom making a diagnosis is impossible. In such cases it is extremely difficult to manage the pain experienced.

Deformity

Due to contracture formation (see page 14), or to previous disease, the hip can become very deformed. This can make walking impossible and hip replacement may be offered as treatment in such cases. However, it is rare to replace a hip for reasons of deformity alone. Patients with deformed hip joints usually also experience pain and it is the presence of the pain in addition to the deformity that justifies the total hip replacement. To perform the operation for deformity alone can be successful in terms of range of movement and function, but may leave a disappointed patient. This is because the term hip 'replacement' is slightly incorrect. The operation does not provide a true replacement hip; the end result is an *artificial* hip. Consequently, after surgery, patients frequently feel slight discomfort within the hip joint. Also, to expect an artificial hip to behave exactly like a normal one would is unrealistic. This sometimes happens, but not always.

The Other Joints Need to be Protected

When hip disease is fairly well advanced, it is possible for the joint to become so destroyed that pain diminishes. As destruction progresses, so the range of movement decreases and so the strains normally borne by the hip are taken up by the joints surrounding it – in particular, the knee and spine (see Chapter 3). It is occasionally necessary to perform a hip replacement in order to protect these adjacent joints from further damage. Patients with longstanding hip deformity due, for example, to a childhood infection, can walk for many years in an odd manner and eventually damage the spine or the knee. Should this occur, then hip replacement can help relieve pain and give protection to the surrounding joints.

The Causes of Pain, Deformity and Stress on Nearby Joints

These three indications for hip replacement considered above can be caused by a variety of diseases. It is these diseases that will now be described.

OSTEOARTHRITIS

Osteoarthritis (see Figure 4.1) is a disease of the articular cartilage of certain joints. Not all joints are affected by it, but it can, none the less, be pretty widespread in any one patient.

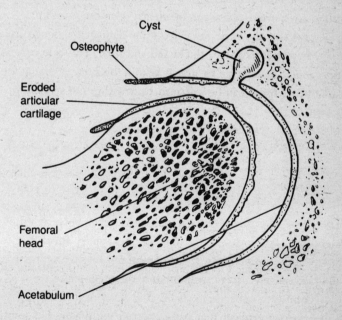

Figure 4.1 *Diagrammatic representation of an osteoarthritic hip joint.*

It is not a new condition. Not only has it been found that primitive man suffered from osteoarthritis, but it can also be seen throughout the animal kingdom, in birds and even dinosaurs.

As we get older, so the incidence of the disease increases, with more than 50 per cent of people over the age of 40 experiencing degenerative changes in the weight-bearing joints. In the early stages of osteoarthritis, there are changes within the articular cartilage that lead to its flaking and damage. The body attempts to repair these damaged areas and, in the process of doing so, can produce too much cartilage. Blood flow to the affected area is increased as the body does this and the extra bits of cartilage are transformed into bony lips, called *osteophytes*. These can be clearly seen on X-rays.

Eventually, the bone underlying the damaged articular cartilage becomes exposed, thickened and hard. This is known as *eburnation*. Cysts begin to appear within this bone while, at the same time, there can be inflammation within the synovium – *synovitis*.

There are two basic forms of osteoarthritis:

- primary
- secondary.

The cause of primary osteoarthritis has never been definitely identified, but it tends to start in the hands, spreading to involve other joints later. It can sometimes be very aggressive, and particularly affects women after the menopause.

Secondary osteoarthritis is created as a result of some previous disease process that has occurred within the hip joint, such as an old infection, a birth defect or an old injury. Dislocations of the hip joint, though relatively uncommon, are frequently associated with later onset of osteoarthritis. Other rare causes of osteoarthritis include certain conditions of the nervous system (for example, syphilis), localized areas of bone death (such as that which may happen after someone has experienced the 'bends' or after alcoholism, long-term steroid use or long-term use of certain anti-inflammatory drugs), disorders of the body's metabolism (say, gout) and nutritional disorders (such as certain fungi found in Siberia and Northern China). The list is endless.

The progression of osteoarthritis can be hastened where a person who has it is overweight. This is because the heavier you are, the greater the stress passing through the weight-bearing joints is and the more likely it is that osteoarthritis will both develop and progress once established. The symptoms may appear more significant at damper, colder times of year.

The Management of Osteoarthritis

The management of osteoarthritis, as with many other conditions, can be achieved by either medical or surgical means. Patients can do much to help themselves and avoid the need for medical help at all in the early stages. Losing excess weight, taking regular exercise and making certain changes at work and to your lifestyle can all be very beneficial. However, despite such efforts, it is likely that treatment will eventually be needed.

In the early stages, the only medical treatment that will be required is the taking of simple painkillers (*analgesics*), such as paracetamol. There comes a time, though, when such painkillers alone are insufficient. At that stage, an anti-inflammatory agent should be offered. The commonest anti-inflammatory medicine is aspirin, but a group of compounds referred to as *non-steroidal anti-inflammatory drugs* (NSAIDs) are also widely used in the treatment of degenerative joint disease. Some NSAIDs do have side-effects and they are not always tolerated by everyone.

While someone is modifying their lifestyle to cope with osteoarthritis, it is worth considering physiotherapy as an aid to treatment. Short courses of a few treatments are perhaps better than long courses over protracted periods. Hydrotherapy (exercises undertaken in a pool) can also bring some relief from symptoms.

There are many other ways in which you can relieve the pain of an osteoarthritic hip joint. Only a few have been mentioned here, but many have found homeopathy, osteopathy, acupuncture, reflexology, aromatherapy and other paramedical treatments to be beneficial.

Once these milder forms of treatment have reached their limit of success, consideration should be given to injection of the hip joint. Injection may be either into the joint (*intra-articular injection*) or immediately outside it (*peri-articular injection*) (see Chapter 3 for further details of these).

RHEUMATOID ARTHRITIS

Rheumatoid arthritis is a common condition caused by inflammation of the synovium – synovitis. It can affect many joints in the body, often being most painful in the morning, and may result in a generalized feeling of malaise and fatigue. Though commoner in adults, it can also affect children, causing the very distressing condition of *juvenile rheumatoid arthritis*.

One thing I have found is that people with this kind of arthritis are always charming individuals. Also, that the more severe the condition is, the nicer the person seems to be!

Rheumatoid arthritis is a very erosive condition, frequently being associated with thin and fragile bone, something that can make hip replacement technically difficult. There are other causes of synovitis, though rheumatoid arthritis is perhaps the most common, and all of these can erode the bone, eventually meaning that the joint needs to be replaced.

INFECTION

Bone and joint infections can be deep-seated and long-lasting problems. Pus is damaging to articular cartilage and only needs to be in contact with it for a matter of hours before permanent damage can be done. Fortunately, hip joint infection is rare, but before antibiotics were widely used it was commoner. It would frequently affect children who would recover, but whose hip joints were then irreversibly damaged. As children are pretty resilient, they would frequently keep going until 20 to 30 years of age. At that stage, significant osteoarthritis could have set in. In such cases, the surgeon is then faced with the difficult problem of what treatment option should be offered to a young adult with advanced hip disease.

Tuberculosis, a chronic infection, can also cause extensive destruction of the hip. This can occur later in life, though it can affect children, and may also result in subsequent osteoarthritis.

To undertake hip replacement surgery in patients with a previous history of infection is possible, but can be risky. A patient can have no symptoms of residual infection and yet some bacteria can still be present in the hip area. For many years, the patient can be unaware of this fact. If surgery is then performed, the original infection can be reactivated. Precautions are taken at surgery to avoid this happening, but there may be an increased chance of infection following the hip replacement operation when it is performed in such cases.

METABOLIC BONE DISEASE

Abnormalities of the body's metabolism can cause crystals to be deposited within the hip joint. The commonest condition to have this effect is gout, where there is a build-up of urate crystals within articular cartilage. This damages the surface of the joint, osteoarthritis being the eventual result. If diagnosed early, gout can frequently be controlled with medicines. However, should it advance to the stage where joint damage occurs, a hip replacement may be the only option.

FRACTURES

Fractures can affect all age groups for a variety of reasons. However, particularly in the elderly, fractures around the hip joint are common. The fracture often occurs across the femoral neck and, as it does so, can disrupt the blood supply to the femoral head. Once the blood supply has been disrupted, the femoral head can die and the natural hip joint be destroyed. This is not truly osteoarthritis, but, rather, is referred to as *avascular necrosis*. The effect on the patient, however, is the same in both cases. The hip becomes painful, deformed and mobility is dramatically reduced. Hip replacement is therefore frequently recommended in such cases. This may be in the form of a hemiarthroplasty or a total hip replacement (see Chapter 3).

The advantage of a hip replacement for people who have suffered fractures, be it hemiarthroplasty or total replacement, is that it allows them to be mobile again very soon after surgery. In certain circumstances an attempt is made to fix the fracture, rather than to replace the hip. This is an excellent idea provided the fracture heals. Unfortunately, in some people, the fracture does not heal because of the damage to the blood supply that occurred at the time of the injury. There is therefore an argument for replacing the hip joint in *all* patients who have had a fracture across the femoral neck, and certainly whenever the fracture is severely displaced, that is, when the two broken ends of the bone have moved quite far apart.

Unfortunately, where a hip replacement is given for a

fractured femoral neck, the results may not be as good as when the replacement is performed due to osteoarthritis. This may be because prior to the fracture, the patient had no pain. There had not been the long period of unrelenting discomfort that is associated with the osteoarthritic hip and the relief the replacement hip then brings from that pain. A patient who was completely normal before they fractured their hip, quite justifiably, wishes to be completely normal afterwards, but a hip replacement, however good it may be, cannot always provide such a level of confidence.

It is sometimes necessary to perform a total hip replacement to prevent a fracture from occurring. Certain conditions are associated with the development of *stress fractures* of the upper femur. A stress fracture is a tiny break in one edge of the femur, usually in bone that is abnormal in composition. Such a break has not fully extended across the femur to become a complete fracture. If this is noticed in time, then a hip replacement is sometimes performed in order to splint the stress fracture and prevent the break from extending across the bone. The commonest condition causing such a fracture for which a hip replacement is performed is known as *Paget's disease*, a disease that affects the structure of bone and can lead to significant bowing and bending of the lower limbs.

TUMOURS

As with many other tissues, bone can be the site of tumours. These are sometimes benign (harmless), sometimes malignant (likely to cause harm). The malignant tumours can arise directly from the bone itself (*primary tumours*) or occur as a result of the spread of a tumour or tumours elsewhere in the body (*secondary tumours*).

The presence of a bone tumour within the upper femur causes weakness of the bone and may increase the risk of the bone fracturing. If such a risk exists, hip replacement is frequently offered. As with Paget's disease, the weak point is splinted and the possibility of fracture is removed. Also, for certain malignant tumours, total hip replacement makes it possible to remove the tumour while the hip replacement operation is being carried out. This can be a very effective method for controlling pain.

NEUROLOGICAL CONDITIONS

Certain neurological conditions – essentially, diseases of the nervous system – can cause damage to the hip joint. This is thought to be because the damaged nerves no longer allow the person to feel pain. As a result, damage can occur to the joint without that person realizing it. In such circumstances, osteoarthritic change can be very rapid and aggressive.

Total hip replacement in such cases is fraught with problems. Because the patient is unaware of the problems occurring in the hip joint, they will also be unaware of problems arising within a *replacement* hip joint. Where such damage has occurred, such joints are referred to as *neuropathic* joints, or *Charcot* joints, and replacements of them are only rarely indicated because of the problems involved in replacing them.

5

DESIGNS OF HIP REPLACEMENT

It is remarkable that, for an operation that is so widely performed and for which results are predictable, there are so many different designs of total hip replacement. Worldwide, there are thousands of different types and, for each one, there is someone claiming that their design is the best. It would be impossible to list here all the designs available, but there are certain principles that apply to a successful design. From time to time the media will report on the creation of a 'new' design of total hip replacement – the replacement that will ostensibly last forever and avoid the problems experienced by so many other hip replacements – but only very rarely are the long-term results of these designs given equal press attention.

This situation is compounded by the fact that no legislation exists to set out what the 'standard' total hip replacement should be. Legislation does exist limiting the nature of the materials that can be used, but not the design the joint should conform to. For example, it would be perfectly possible for me to design a total hip replacement on the back of an envelope, find an engineering company to make it for me and then insert it into a patient the following week. Provided the materials from which that hip replacement was made were the recognized, safe materials, then this would be perfectly legal. It is therefore worth stopping to consider the whole subject of the replacement hip itself, how designs have changed over the years and why they have changed. The aim of the 'perfect' total hip replacement is to remain fixed to the patient's bone for the rest of time. If this situation could be truly achieved, then no hip replacement would ever fail and each operation would last for life. This is manifestly not the case and it is for this reason that so many designs now exist — each design seeks to achieve perfection.

The Terminology

As with the human body, the components of total hip replacements can be described in anatomical terms. The thigh bone component is referred to as the *femoral* component. It may have a *stem* that is inserted down the shaft of the femur. At its top end is the ball-like *head*. The head is joined to the stem by the *neck*, the junction between neck and stem being called the *shoulder*. At the shoulder there is sometimes to be found a *collar* that rests on the patient's divided femoral neck. The acetabular component is sometimes referred to as the *cup* or *socket*. The back of the acetabular component is the part that is in contact with the patient's own acetabular bone.

Sometimes, rather than using the word 'component', surgeons will use the word 'prosthesis'. The two terms mean the same and can be used interchangeably, for both acetabular and femoral components.

How the Replacement Hip is Fixed to the Bone

Two methods of fixing the replacement component to the bone are used to achieve the best bond between the two:

- cemented
- uncemented (sometimes referred to as *cementless*).

Both methods have their protagonists and critics. The decision as to which method is used depends very much on the surgeon concerned and the country in which the patient lives. For example, the use of cementless components is widespread on mainland Europe, but is less widespread in the United Kingdom.

Orthopaedic trends have much to do with which method is used. Some years the cementless design will appear to be in favour, while in others the cemented designs will be more commonly used. Often such decisions are based on the appearance in the orthopaedic literature of the poor results achieved when one or the other design has been used. More logic is now being applied, but it will be many years before it is truly known which method is better than the other.

THE CEMENTED METHOD

Perhaps the most significant advance in orthopaedic surgery this century was when John Charnley proposed that the femoral and acetabular components be secured to a patient's bone with cement. The cement he suggested was known as *polymethylmethacrylate* (PMMA). In the mid 1950s, when he was undertaking his research, this was a state of the art cement. It was being considered by the dental profession as a

filling material and it is to John Charnley's credit that he dared
to use it in a patient and to show that it would work. In fact,
it is said that John Charnley was not the first person to use
polymethylmethacrylate cement to secure a total hip replacement. However, he was unquestionably the first to demonstrate that it could be used successfully in this situation and to
scientifically prove its efficiency.

The cement acts like grout in that it is not used as a glue,
but a space filler. When a hole is prepared in either the
patient's acetabulum or femoral shaft, this may be filled with
cement, allowing the component to be inserted and held in
position until the cement has set. Around the prosthesis is
then created a secure cement *mantle* (see Figure 5.1).

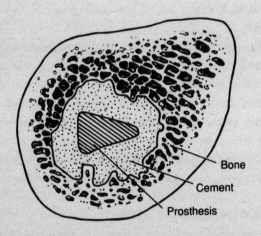

Bone

Cement

Prosthesis

Figure 5.1 *Cross-section of a portion of a femur, showing cement inter-
locking with the patient's own bone for a tight, secure bonding of component
and bone.*

Polymethylmethacrylate, though highly successful as an orthopaedic cement, is perceived by some as being an outdated one. Indeed, most dentists no longer consider using it as a filling material, because of its poor performance when compared with more modern cements. Much work has therefore been done to try and develop new orthopaedic cements. None of the cements this work has proposed has really become established in the marketplace today, though, and so polymethylmethacrylate still continues to be the cement of choice.

Dentists widely use composite resins. Composite resins are cements that contain tiny pieces of a chosen solid, allowing the cement to be given mechanical properties similar to those of the living tissue to which it is attached. When a force is applied to the cement, such as might happen when a prosthesis is held in place by it and the person walks and so on, there is little differential movement between the cement and the surrounding living tissue. This may prolong the life of the prosthesis/cement complex. Composite resins have been tried instead of the traditional cement, but they are expensive and have not become widely used.

Other types of cement are more closely related to polymethylmethacrylate. Polymethylmethacrylate is used in industry, under pressure, to make Perspex. There is nothing else mixed into it and it is therefore known as an unfilled resin. Another unfilled resin that has been used in orthopaedic surgery is *butylmethacrylate*. This did not perform as well as polymethylmethacrylate and so did not continue to be used.

Polymethylmethacrylate

Polymethylmethacrylate comes in a variety of forms. At its most basic it consists of a liquid and a powder that are mixed together by hand or mechanically. Within minutes, the mixture has set hard (or *cured*).

As the mechanical properties of a metal prosthesis are different to those of the surrounding bone, it is impossible for polymethylmethacrylate to behave in the same way where it comes into contact with the metal component as it does where it is in contact with bone. It is therefore a material of compromise, doing the best it can to fill the gap between the two.

Recognizing that polymethylmethacrylate is a compromise material, orthopaedic manufacturers have, on occasion, coated the metal stem of the femoral component with polymethylmethacrylate prior to surgery. This is referred to as *precoating* and allows for a good bond between the polymethylmethacrylate and the metal stem.

Though polymethylmethacrylate is widely used, surgeons have for a long time been concerned about the presence of such an extra element in a hip replacement. The use of cement introduces another point of failure within the hip replacement complex. If a hip does fail, and the femoral component needs to be removed, there is a barrier of cement still left within the shaft of the femur that must be extracted. This is not an easy task.

When polymethylmethacrylate is used to fix an acetabular component in place, it is sometimes possible for pieces of cement to bulge into the pelvis and to damage underlying soft tissue structures. Polymethylmethacrylate, then, has advantages, but is not problem-free.

THE CEMENTLESS METHOD

Due to concern about the use of cement and the difficulties it can sometimes create, cementless components have been designed. Indeed, in the early days of total hip replacement, cementless components were quite common.

The logic of performing a cementless operation is that it can be quicker to undertake and might avoid the problems associated with having to remove cement during a subsequent revision operation. It also eliminates one of the things that can possibly go wrong after hip surgery.

Because no cement layer is used in the cementless method, much energy has been expended on finding the ideal surface for the component, one into which a patient's bone can grow. The objective, then, is to provide a 'bone-friendly' surface that will, in time, become so securely knitted with the patient's own bone that loosening at the prosthesis/bone junction will be impossible.

In the early days of cementless components, simple stainless steel was used. The polished surface meant that very little integration between bone and prosthesis could occur. A blasted surface was then used, the roughened surface providing more grip for the bone tissue. Holes and irregularities were then built into the components, screws to fix them to the bone introduced, and even whole femoral stems that screwed down into the shaft of the femur appeared. Surgery involving such designs was sometimes a formidable undertaking.

However, though the logic behind such designs is sound, the results rarely competed with the recognized performance of designs fixed using the cemented method. Generally, the long-term results of cementless designs have not surpassed the long-term results of cemented ones. Other modifications of the surface of the prosthesis have therefore been considered. Covering the surface of the components with tiny metal beads – a process known as *porous coating* – was said to encourage the bone to attach itself to the metal surface (see Figure 5.2). Some evidence exists that this actually occurs, but, so far, it is confined to a handful of cases, despite the widespread use in the 1990s of porous-coated components.

A more modern innovation is the development of a material called hydroxyapatite (see Figure 5.3). This is one of

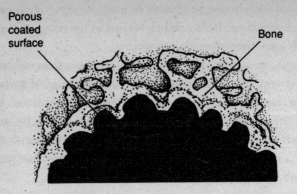

Figure 5.2 *Bone growing into a porous-coated surface. It is unusual to find bone in contact with every nook and cranny.*

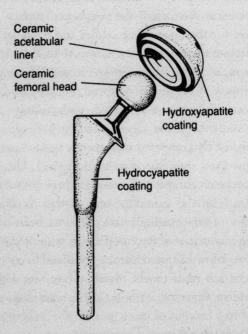

Figure 5.3 *A modular, hydroxyapatite-coated hip replacement. Note the ceramic head and acetabulum, designed to reduce the quantity of wear debris produced by the bearing surface.*

the body's own chemicals within bone. Coating a prosthesis with hydroxyapatite therefore allows excellent ingrowth of bone into the hydroxyapatite coating. There is scientific research to support this concept. However, a point of failure is now recognized to exist, that of the junction between the hydroxyapatite and prosthesis. However well the bone knits with the hydroxyapatite, the material does not necessarily maintain a long-term bond with the prosthesis itself. Early results suggest that hydroxyapatite coating might be as good as cemented replacement hips in the short term, but how they will behave in the long term is still unknown.

HYBRID TOTAL HIP REPLACEMENT

Neither cemented nor cementless methods are perfect. For this reason, many surgeons have considered the use of a mixture of the two, hence the *hybrid* total hip replacement.

The motivating principle behind the hybrid total hip replacement is that the long-term results of the cementless femoral components may not be as good as the long-term results of the cemented ones. Also, the long-term results of the cemented acetabular components are not always as good as the cementless ones. So, some have suggested using a cementless acetabular component and a cemented femoral component. Logically this should improve the results of hip replacements and, at the time of writing, there is scientific research to show that the results of the hybrid total hip replacement after six and a half years are as good as those of a totally cemented hip replacement. What the results will be in the longer term, however, we will have to wait to see.

The Criteria that Influence the Choice of Replacement Hip

With so many designs on the market, both cemented and cementless, how does an orthopaedic surgeon decide which hip replacement is suitable for a patient? Although surgeons will generally remain faithful to a limited number of designs that they know can be inserted safely and have been successful in the past, which is chosen for any one patient will be influenced in part by a surgeon's training and in part by what is easily available in their local area. In short, it must be a prosthesis that the surgeon knows they can insert safely and has a history of good results.

Beyond these criteria, a surgeon may often decide to use a cementless design if it is likely that a revision operation will be needed in the future. As it is currently felt that it is impossible to make all hip replacements last for life, the younger the person, the more likely it is that a revision operation will be needed. Many surgeons, therefore, opt for a cementless design for younger people and cemented ones for the elderly.

Femoral Component Design

When John Charnley first pioneered his total hip replacement, the prosthetic femoral stem was straight. At the same time, other surgeons, particularly in mainland Europe, were proposing a stem with a different shape. This was a curved stem, frequently referred to as a *banana stem*.

The banana stem became popular because it was easier to insert during the operation. Certain surgical approaches performed during a hip replacement operation do not allow the surgeon to look straight down the femur, thereby making it very difficult to insert a straight stem. The banana stem was easier to use in such situations. However, it has now largely disappeared because the results, though sometimes good, were not uniformly successful. The majority of femoral stems used today are therefore straight, just as Charnley originally suggested.

If you look at cross-sections of femoral stems, they may be either sharp or rounded. The banana stems were largely sharp, though it soon became apparent that the sharpened borders placed significant stress on the mantle of cement that surrounded the component, which resulted in cement failure. Smooth edges and rounded borders were therefore introduced and most stems used today retain these features to avoid the problem of cement failure.

At the point where the neck and stem of the femoral component meet, a *collar* can sometimes be found. Collars were a widespread design feature in the early days of total hip replacement, though they are less commonly seen now. The logic of the collar was that it gave added support to the femoral component as it rested on the patient's own transected femoral neck. However, it was found that this did not happen in practice. What the collar did was transfer the stresses of movement in a way that the body would not do naturally, which caused certain areas of the patient's own bone to disappear. Collars are therefore not widely used today, but some new designs still appear that do feature collars none the less.

The length of femoral stem varies a lot. Some are very long, some are short. There is little long-term work to show that any one particular length of stem is ideal. In cementless designs, the stem tends to be longer than it does in cemented designs. This provides a greater surface area for the bone to knit to. In cemented designs, however, this would be a disadvantage as the longer the stem, the further down the shaft of the femur the cement mantle will extend, which can cause considerable problems during revision surgery.

The kind of surface the femoral component has is also variable. The different kinds of surfaces cementless designs can have were discussed on pages 45 – 7, but there are various options for cemented designs too. There are two schools of thought on the matter. One says that the stem should have a blasted, irregular surface to allow the cement to bond well with it. However, this does not take into account the fact that femoral components subside with time. This subsidence occurs at the junction between the cement and prosthetic stem. Some designs of cemented component therefore have a polished surface, which allows the femoral component to gradually subside within the cement mantle without disrupting the cement itself.

At the top end of the femoral component can be found the femoral head. This is colloquially referred to as the *ball*. Different ball diameters are available. In Charnley's design, the ball size was slightly more than 22 mm (approximately ⅞ in). He introduced this size because he felt that it would reduce the amount of friction created when the hip joint was working. At the same time, others were proposing that a 32 mm (approximately 1¼ in) ball size was appropriate.

For a long time, orthopaedic surgeons used *either* the 22 mm ball *or* the 32 mm one. Opinion then changed, surgeons thinking that the two available sizes represented extremes and a compromise situation would be better. Thus, the 28 mm (about 1⅛ in) ball was introduced. This is perhaps the most widely used ball diameter today, but other diameters do exist.

Modularity of design is a more recent trend. Modularity means that a femoral component is no longer made as one complete piece: the ball may be separate from the neck, which, in turn, may be separate from the stem. Stem length can also be modified depending on the needs of the patient.

Modularity has many advantages, including the fact that the surgeon can 'build' a total hip replacement at the time of the operation in order that the new hip can be matched to the patient as closely as possible. However, whenever there is a junction between two pieces of metal, *fretting* (wear caused by the parts rubbing) can occur and this can happen with modular designs.

Modularity, therefore, though good, is not a perfect solution. Despite this, many femoral components used today do have a modular ball. This allows it to be attached to the neck at the end of the operation, which optimizes hip stability.

Acetabular Component Design

If one talks to an orthopaedic surgeon about hip replacement design, almost immediately conversation will turn to the femoral component. The acetabular component, important though it is, always appears to draw less attention. None the less, acetabular component failure is often the first thing to happen when a hip replacement begins to loosen. Certain basic principles of design have been considered over the years, but more work still needs to be undertaken to ensure perfection.

One of the acetabular components initially proposed by Charnley was made of Teflon. This appeared to be an excellent material, but it rapidly became apparent that it wore away too quickly. For this reason, a special type of polyethylene was introduced – *high-density polyethylene* (HDPE). This is the material used for most acetabular components worldwide today.

In its early days, the HDPE used for acetabular design was thin. This did not apply to the Charnley acetabular component, where the HDPE layer was significantly thicker. Charnley's recommendation that a thicker layer be used proved to be correct. The thicker the acetabular component, within limits, the longer the component is likely to last. It is believed that this is because the component changes shape due to the stresses imposed on it during walking. The change is only slight, but the thinner the plastic, the more it changes. The more it changes, the greater is the stress that is applied to the surrounding cement mantle, which speeds up any subsequent loosening. Thicker HDPE cups are now recommended to avoid this happening.

There was a phase in orthopaedic surgery during which it was felt that the HDPE cup should have a metal backing. It was believed that this would significantly strengthen the component and thereby prevent loosening. Metal backing was to be used in conjunction with cement. In practice, however, this theory did not appear to hold true. Metal-backed components have been shown to sometimes fail *earlier* than the simple HDPE designs and so they are no longer used in many orthopaedic centres.

For cemented designs, it is important to ensure that there is an even mantle of cement around the acetabular component during the cementing process. Many components have small studs on the back to ensure that the cement mantle applied is of an even thickness. As the surgeon pushes the cup into the cement-filled acetabular cavity, the studs prevent the cup from coming into direct contact with the patient's bone, it remaining separated from it by the cement mantle.

The acetabular component has not escaped modularity either, particularly the cementless designs. These depend on a metal backing that is frequently porous-coated (see page 45). Metal backing appears to be a problem with cemented acetabular components, but not necessarily with the cementless designs. The backing is inserted first against the patient's own bone. Once the component is securely in place, an HDPE liner is introduced. This liner can be of varying thickness and diameter with special features built in that allow maximum stability of the hip joint.

The Bearing Surface

This is the point of contact between ball and cup. It is the behaviour of this surface that largely determines the success or failure of the hip replacement.

However smooth the bearing surface is, there will always be some friction. This friction creates small particles of bearing material, referred to as *wear debris*. It is now known that the production of wear debris plays a significant part in the eventual loosening of a total hip replacement. The debris sets up a low-grade inflammatory reaction that, in turn, causes the patient's bone to become absorbed. This process is known as *osteolysis*. Much time and effort has therefore been expended in trying to reduce the wear debris produced by a total hip replacement. Special metals, and special plastics, have been tried and tested.

In the early days of total hip replacement a metal-to-metal joint was used – a large-diameter metal ball was inserted into an equally large-diameter metal acetabular cup. Some did well, but the production of metal debris was often dramatic and, occasionally, the metal-to-metal joint would even seize up, no longer being able to move.

This phenomenon led Charnley to devise a metal-on-Teflon design. Further developments led to the metal-on-HDPE design. However, even metal-on-HDPE has been shown to produce significant debris and other materials have therefore been introduced. A ceramic surface was considered – a ceramic ball and a ceramic cup – but this was very expensive and technically difficult to use, though friction was reduced significantly. The wear debris produced was minimal, but only if the ceramic surface remained undamaged – as soon as it was damaged (which could happen during the operation itself), then the joint produced a significant amount of wear debris.

A ceramic-on-HDPE joint was the next development. This provided a cheaper alternative to the ceramic-on-ceramic design and friction was less than in the metal-on-HDPE design. The ceramic-on-HDPE option is still widely used today by surgeons who wish to lower the production of wear debris, but who do not want to make the operation too expensive. Different varieties of HDPE are being introduced in order to reduce wear debris production still further. Also, different metals have been used for the ball.

Frequently, the femoral stem will be made either of stainless steel or of titanium. When titanium was first used it was also used as a bearing surface for the ball. However, it was found that when titanium was used as a bearing surface, it did not withstand the rigours of time. It wore away rapidly, became deformed and was associated with the production of significant quantities of wear debris. It has therefore been largely abandoned as a bearing surface material, being replaced by metal alloys, in particular cobalt-chrome. Indeed, the commonest ball materials used today are cobalt-chrome or ceramic ones.

The situation is confused further by still more research. Because of the problems associated with wear debris, a metal-to-metal joint is being reconsidered once again. The wheel, it could be said, has almost turned a full circle. The thinking is that metal-to-metal designs failed in the past due to the comparitively poorer engineering facilities available at that time. Now, with precision engineering being possible, exact matches between ball and cup size can be obtained. The metal-to-metal option has thus returned and may be *the* option for many years to come.

Other Designs

Surgeons have long been concerned about the amount of bone that needs to be removed during a total hip replacement operation. The less bone that is removed, the better it is for the patient and the greater are the chances that any revision operation that is necessary in the years to come will be successful.

In 1939, Smith-Petersen introduced his interposition arthroplasty, a design of surface replacement of the hip (see page 25). This replacement involved fixing a small cup, rather like a contraceptive diaphragm, to the top of the femoral head. Again, the wheel appears to have come full circle, with surface replacement now returning as an operation of choice in certain orthopaedic centres. It allows limited bone resection, which means that a minimal amount of bone is removed, making it particularly suitable for younger patients, though long-term results are still not available.

A compromise situation was introduced in the late 1980s when a femoral component was developed, the insertion of which involved limited resection of the patient's femoral neck. This again preserved more of the patient's bone, thereby leaving more natural tissue to support the artificial femoral component.

Though a sensible and logical design, the operation proved difficult for many surgeons and so the procedure never became widely established. The long-term results of this design are still awaited.

As was discussed in Chapter 3, in the early days of hip replacement, it was considered necessary only to replace the femoral side of the joint – a hemiarthroplasty. Such an operation then went out of favour, being mainly reserved for the management of fractures in the hip area. However, even today, there are some surgeons who undertake hemiarthroplasty for osteoarthritis. The results are not as good as those that can be expected for a fully cemented design, but they can be improved by the addition to the femoral component of an articulated acetabular component, where the femoral and acetabular components come as one piece. This is known as a *bipolar* replacement and has had useful short-term results. The long-term results do not always appear to be able to challenge those of a standard cemented design. None the less, they are still widely used in certain centres.

Just as bespoke clothing fits better than off-the-peg garments, surgeons and designers have thought that if a purpose-made hip replacement, specifically designed for the patient, were inserted that this would ensure the greatest longevity of the replacement. These are known as *custom* components and are used in many centres worldwide today. However, they are expensive and, defying the logic, their long-term results do not appear to surpass those of the standard designs as yet. Long-term results, in large numbers, are still awaited.

Revision Hip Replacements

The above comments apply to primary hip replacements. The technical problems that face the surgeon performing revision surgery, though, are very different to those encountered the first time. The patient will already have a primary hip replacement in place, the operation often having been performed a number of years ago. Often, too, there is extensive loss of the patient's own natural bone, infection may be present, fractures may have occurred and . . . the list continues. Thus, special components now exist to assist the revision hip surgeon. Longer stems are available, greater modularity can be obtained, reinforcement rings assist with strengthening the acetabular component and wire meshes exist to support both acetabulum and femur. Cemented and uncemented designs are available and the points made in this chapter regarding both types also apply to components used in revision surgery. Unfortunately, the main difference between primary and revision surgery is that it is harder to achieve a satisfactory result with a revision replacement than it is with the primary procedure.

6

PRIMARY HIP REPLACEMENT – THE OPERATION

Once the decision has been taken to perform a total hip replacement, it is not just a matter of turning up on the day and allowing everything to happen. What occurs pre-operatively, and immediately post-operatively, is as important as the operation itself.

The first step for the surgeon is to ensure that the patient is as fit as possible medically, so that they are able to withstand the rigours of surgery. However successful the operation may be, the whole experience is stressful for the patient and not all complications associated with surgery are directly related to the operation itself. Following a hip operation, it is possible for the hip replacement to be functioning well, but for the cardiovascular system to malfunction or the gastrointestinal tract to fail. An overall assessment prior to surgery is therefore important, looking at *all* the body's systems, not just the musculoskeletal one.

Pre-operative Assessment

To assist in assessing the condition of the patient as a whole, many surgeons run pre-operative assessment clinics. There may also be an associated anaesthetic assessment clinic where more severe non-surgical problems are considered.

Visits to the clinics are arranged several weeks before surgery and allow a thorough check on the patient's overall state of health to be carried out beforehand. Sufficient time should be allowed between the visit to the clinic and the operation to enable further investigations and corrections to be made if they are necessary. Even if a *formal* pre-operative assessment does not take place, it is sensible for patients to be seen at least two weeks prior to the operation so that everything is ready on the day.

The kinds of checks included in a pre-operative assessment vary, but the commonest are described below.

HAEMOGLOBIN LEVEL

The blood is tested to see whether or not its oxygen-carrying capacity is sufficient, which is measured by seeing how much haemoglobin it contains. There is always blood loss, during and after the operation, and if the haemoglobin starts at a low level before surgery it may eventually fall far enough to pose a risk to the patient. A low haemoglobin level also makes patients feel very lethargic after surgery and delays their recovery from it.

BLOOD CROSS-MATCHING

Approximately 30 per cent of patients will require blood transfusion after a hip replacement operation. The average blood loss, taking operative and post-operative volumes into account, is slightly more than 1 litre (1¼ pints). Blood should therefore be cross-matched and ready for the operation. Sometimes patients can have unusual antibodies within their own blood, making an accurate cross-match difficult. It is unwise to proceed with a hip replacement if there is no appropriate blood available.

ELECTROCARDIOGRAM (ECG)

This is a simple assessment of how healthy the heart is. Hip replacements are frequently given to those over the age of 60, many of whom have had heart problems or are developing such problems without realizing it. The heart must be strong enough to withstand the stress of surgery. However, the existence of a weak cardiovascular system does not necessarily mean that surgery has to be avoided. It is possible, in some centres, for patients with very weak hearts to receive a hip replacement. However, it is important that both anaesthetist and surgeon are forewarned of any problems, so that appropriate therapies can be given to support the heart during and after surgery.

UREA AND ELECTROLYTE ESTIMATION

This is an investigation that provides a brief overview of the body's biochemistry. For a period after surgery, particularly in the elderly, it is possible for biochemical control to be significantly impaired. Correct levels may be maintained with appropriate medicines, including intravenous drips. However, it is important that everyone knows the baseline level at which the patient starts. Also, it can be hazardous to undertake surgery when the blood levels of certain chemicals are outside the normal range. This particularly applies to the body's potassium level.

URINE TESTING

A simple ward test of a patient's urine is a vital part of pre-operative assessment. Many elderly patients have longstanding urinary tract infections but are totally unaware of them. Knowing about any infections is important because there is a significant link between urinary tract infections and infected joint replacements. Thus, any infections need to be identified and treated before surgery is undertaken.

X-RAYS (RADIOGRAPHS, ROENTGENOGRAMS)

A chest X-ray is usually given to elderly patients as it is useful to look at this together with the results of the ECG. Troubles within the chest, of which the patient may be unaware, can then be identified. These can be treated before surgery, if necessary, or after the operation.

A further hip X-ray may also be performed at this stage. In certain countries, there is a long waiting list for hip replacement and so sometimes more than a year can have elapsed since the patient was first seen in the out-patient department. During this time, the severity of hip disease, and the deformity associated with it, can change, so an updated X-ray is necessary in order that the surgeon can make the right decisions.

OTHER TESTS

Though the above tests are what the majority of patients will need to have done, certain patients will require other investigations that relate to their specific situation. For example, an alcoholic will need to receive liver function tests, a drug addict an HIV test and patients on certain medical therapies may need to have further blood tests to establish what levels of the drugs are in their bloodstream.

Not only is it important for a patient to be investigated pre-operatively for problems that may influence the operation, but it is also vital that thought be given to what is going to happen when they go home after surgery, 10 to 14 days later. For example, is it necessary to book a room in a convalescent home? Who is going to do the shopping for the first week or 10 days after they return home? Is there any need for specific appliances in the home to make life easier after a hip replacement?

Thought should be given to what will happen and what arrangements will be necessary. The surgeon, physiotherapist, occupational therapist, certain charities and your doctor should all be able to provide sound advice relevant to each person's particular situation.

On Admission

For most units, the day of admission is the day immediately before the operation. Certain patients may be admitted earlier, though, if final tests and readjustments need to be made. For example, some patients take long-term anticoagulant treatment for cardiovascular problems and it is often necessary for them to reduce their dosage during the time up to and after their operation. Such a patient may come to hospital earlier than normal so that the dosage reduction can be monitored.

On admission, the patient is likely to receive a detailed briefing on the nursing aspects of the care they will receive from nursing staff, together with some initial instruction from a physiotherapist. How to walk with crutches is not something that everyone easily masters and, in any case, it is easier to be given advice on how to use them, or a walking frame, before the operation than afterwards.

The day before surgery, though sometimes on the day of surgery itself, the patient is likely to be seen by the operating surgeon. This is an opportunity for both surgeon and patient to ask further questions of each other. The anaesthetist may also see the patient the day before surgery. This pre-operative visit provides an opportunity to discuss the anaesthetic options available, as hip replacement can be performed using a variety of general or local anaesthetic techniques. At this stage, the results of all the investigations should be available, as well as most of the important aspects of the patient's medical history. The anaesthetist is likely to be particularly interested in any previous operations and anaesthetics experienced, especially if there were any complications. It is also very important to find out if the patient has any allergies. Then any troublesome drugs, antiseptics and dressings can be avoided.

Pre-medication is also considered at this meeting, that is, the administration of one or more drugs a short while before the patient is brought to the operating theatre. Traditionally this used to be given by injection and consisted of a strong, pain-relieving drug (*analgesic*) and another with antisickness and secretion-reducing properties. More recently, drugs with a sedative or tranquillizing effect have been used, and these are as effective when they are given by mouth as they are when they are given in the form of an injection. With the increasing use of daycase surgery (not yet for hip replacement!), it has been shown that the ease with which general anaesthesia can be given and the safety of it is good, even if no formal pre-medication is used. The relevant drugs are given in the anaesthetic room at the same time as the induction of anaesthesia.

The anaesthetist's views can always be asked for when the patient is seen pre-operatively, as well as information about all other aspects of the proposed anaesthetic.

In some units, the area where the surgeon will be operating will be shaved on the day of admission. This is to ensure that the surgical incision takes place in an area of skin that is as clean and sterile as possible. Shaving used to be widely performed, though it is less common to do this now.

There are certain practical difficulties involved when the person being operated on is very hairy. A number of the sticky surgical drapes that are used do not stick to such patients very well. If shaving is not performed on the day of admission, it may be undertaken during the operation itself, as a means of ensuring that the drapes form an effective seal around the area of the incision.

Some surgeons believe that shaving actually increases the chance of infection by releasing bacteria that live on the skin. There is some evidence to support this, so do not be surprised if your surgeon decides that shaving is not for you.

There is a common association between hip replacement and a condition known as *deep vein thrombosis* (DVT). This is when blood clots form within the veins of the legs. In itself, the formation of a DVT can be debilitating, but it may also lead to the life-threatening condition of *pulmonary embolism*.

This will be discussed in more detail later, but save to say here that the risk of this happening should be avoided at all costs. Patients are therefore frequently placed on some form of preventative treatment for DVT. The number of available treatments is vast. At its simplest level, treatment may involve the application of stockings to the legs, while also encouraging the patient to be as mobile and active as possible. Increasingly, though, surgeons are using preparations administered by injection or mouth. These are varieties of anticoagulant treatment given in low doses. Such treatments will often commence immediately prior to surgery.

It is every orthopaedic surgeon's nightmare that a hip replacement will become infected. As a consequence, many surgeons will only perform hip replacement surgery when antibiotics have been administered. There are many different antibiotics, and many different doses, that can be given to a patient to minimize the chances of infection. In certain units, antibiotic therapy will begin the day before the operation, continuing for some time afterwards. The dosage of antibiotics given varies from surgeon to surgeon. Some surgeons give as little as one dose of antibiotics, while others continue with antibiotic treatment for more than a week. There is no common consensus on the length of antibiotic treatment recommended as yet.

The Day of the Operation

Once all the various investigations have been done and the results are considered to be acceptable, the patient is prepared for surgery. Antibiotics and preventative treatment for DVT, if appropriate, are given and the patient is changed into a theatre gown. When the time is right, the patient is taken by trolley from the ward to the operating theatre.

In most modern operating theatres, anaesthetics are administered in an anaesthetic room immediately adjacent to the operating theatre, although in some hospitals anaesthesics are given in the operating theatre itself. The patient is unlikely to be left alone in the anaesthetic room, even for a short period of time. A nurse is usually in attendance, as well as the anaesthetist and an operating theatre technician. It is the job of the operating theatre technician to help the anaesthetist with equipment and drug preparations, while the anaesthetist concentrates specifically on the patient.

The anaesthetist will insert one or more needles into a vein in the arm of the patient. If it proves difficult to find a suitable vein in the arm, one in the feet or even the neck can be used.

Assuming that a general anaesthetic has been chosen, the process of putting a patient to sleep is called *induction*. For this, only a small needle need be used. Once the patient is safely asleep, the anaesthetist will usually give a drug that paralyses the muscles. This enables the anaesthetist to control the patient's breathing throughout the operation, using a breathing tube (*endotracheal tube*) passed through the mouth and into the upper airway (*trachea*). The paralysis also makes it easier for the surgeon to manipulate and dislocate the hip joint during the operation. Controlling the breathing in this way has considerable advantages for the patient. By ensuring that both lungs are well-ventilated, the chances of local underventilation and the development of small, collapsed areas, which can give rise to chest infections in the early days after the operation, are reduced.

The anaesthetist also ensures that one of the inserted needles is the right size to allow any transfusions that may be required to be given. This needle needs to be inserted even if a local anaesthetic technique is used.

Local anaesthesia involves the use of an *epidural*, or *spinal*, injection, which is usually inserted while the patient lies on their side. The process normally takes 10 to 15 minutes to perform and then it takes 15 minutes for the anaesthetic to take effect.

Once asleep, the patient is wheeled by trolley into the operating theatre and lifted on to the operating table. The operating table is a thin, cushioned, but hard table. On its surface there will often be a warming mat to ensure that body temperature is kept as stable as possible throughout the operation. The way in which the patient is positioned on the table will depend on the surgical approach the surgeon wishes to use. For example, the patient may be placed on their side or be laid on their back. Whatever position is chosen, various attachments are used to keep the patient in the same position throughout the operation. This is necessary because it can be dangerous for the patient's position to alter during surgery.

Once the patient has been correctly positioned, the surgeon and those who will assist the surgeon wash their hands. This is referred to as *scrubbing-up*. With the liberal use of antiseptic solution and a scrubbing brush, the surgical team will rigorously wash their hands and arms from fingertips to elbows. They then don sterile operating gowns and sterile operating gloves. Scrubbing-up normally takes place in a small room adjacent to the operating theatre, not in the operating theatre itself.

The surgical team then move from the scrub room into the operating theatre and begin to prepare the patient for surgery.

In certain units, the surgeon will also put on further protective items of clothing at this point. A significant risk in orthopaedic surgery is what is known as *needlestick injury*. Because sharp instruments and saws are used during hip replacement surgery, it is possible that one of the saws will cut a surgeon's glove. As soon as this happens, there is a risk of disease being transmitted from surgeon to patient or from patient to surgeon. Protective barrier gloves may therefore be used and protective eyewear (see Figure 6.1). Also, with the greater awareness about HIV, such protective clothing is now more frequently worn than ever before.

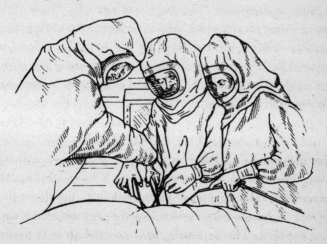

Figure 6.1 *A hip replacement operation. Note the protective equipment worn by the surgical team.*

An orthopaedic operating theatre is not simply a room. To create ideal conditions in order to minimize the chances of infection, a specific kind of air flow is created within it. This is referred to as a *laminar flow*. This means that the direction of air flow over the patient is controlled, ensuring that any bacteria in the theatre air are blown *away* from the patient. Surprisingly enough, all human bodies shed bacteria into the air that surrounds them. Even in the sterile environment of an operating theatre there are bacteria in the air, albeit in low numbers. As it does not take many bacteria to start an infection, laminar flow minimizes the chances of such organisms landing on the patient during surgery. Not all operating theatres have a laminar flow system, as they are very expensive. Where possible, such air flow systems should be used, though, as they can help to reduce infection.

A hip replacement operation involves many different theatre personnel. The surgeon normally has at least one assistant. The anaesthetist also has an operating theatre technician or nurse in attendance. The surgeon is handed instruments by the operating theatre sister, who in turn has a circulating nurse available to help. A minimum of six trained staff are therefore required in the operating theatre in order to undertake a routine total hip replacement. This number does not include staff elsewhere in the operating theatre suite and on the wards.

PREPARATION OF THE PATIENT

The surgeon first applies an antiseptic solution to the area where the incision is to be made. This is to ensure that any bacteria living on the patient's skin are killed. Towels are then applied to the surrounding skin, leaving only the area of incision exposed. This is usually next covered by a thin, see-through plastic drape that adheres directly to the skin. This process is known as *draping*.

Pre-operatively, the surgeon will have decided which operative approach is best for a particular patient. There are many different types of approach, though they fall into three basic categories:

* *anterior*
* *posterior*
* *lateral*.

Orthopaedic surgeons have argued for generations as to which approach is the best. The fact that they are *still* arguing most likely means that it is not the *nature* of the approach that is important. What is vital, though, is that the surgeon knows and understands their own approach intimately and performs it well.

Once the patient has been draped, the incision is made through the see-through plastic layer. Any bleeding that occurs is stopped with an instrument known as a *diathermy*. This applies a small electric current to the blood vessel and cauterizes the bleeding point. The incision is deepened down to the area of the hip joint. Once this area has been reached, the hip is then dislocated.

It is sometimes difficult to dislocate the hip at this point, particularly when the patient has osteoarthritis and it is advanced. Osteophyte formation can be so prolific that they actually prevent dislocation. It can only take place once the osteophytes have been removed. Sometimes, too, the ligamentum teres is so taut that dislocation is impossible. Again, this must be cut to allow dislocation.

Once the hip has been dislocated, the femoral head is exposed. In the osteoarthritic hip, the femoral head looks very knobbly and irregular. The surgeon then takes a special powered saw, often driven by compressed air or battery, and removes the femoral head by dividing the femoral neck. The femoral head is given to the operating theatre sister, who may keep it until the end of the operation. This is in case some bone is needed for grafting at the same time as the hip replacement. Otherwise, some orthopaedic units keep a bone bank — a place where bones are collected and further prepared for use in bone transplantation procedures — so, if the femoral head is not required by the patient for their primary hip replacement, it is sent to the bone bank for use by other patients. This should only be done if the donating patient has given their consent to the hospital.

Once the femoral head has been removed, the acetabulum can be seen beneath it. The soft tissue is removed from the cotyloid fossa and the arthritic cartilage is shaved away. This process is known as *reaming*. Reaming can be performed by hand or using a motorized tool, colloquially known as a *cheese grater*. This is because reamers work rather like a kitchen cheese grater.

The acetabulum is reamed back to healthy-looking bone. It will have been decided pre-operatively whether the patient should have a cemented or cementless acetabular component. If a cemented component is chosen, a number of holes are made in the prepared acetabulum, known as *keyholes*. These are small pits that will enable the cement mantle that will surround the acetabular component to create a good strong bond with the bone.

The raw surface of the acetabulum is then thoroughly washed and dried. While this is being done, the theatre sister will be mixing the bone cement for a cemented component. The cement is inserted into the prepared acetabular cavity and then, normally, it is pressurized. In this way it is possible to ensure high-pressure contact between cement and prepared acetabular bone.

The surgeon then waits until the cement is just beginning to set and, when it is, inserts the cup. It is important that the surgeon does not wait too long! Waiting until the last moment is necessary because the cement needs to be as thick as possible so that when the acetabular cup is inserted, cement is pushed into all the nooks and crannies in the prepared bone and does not flow out again. Then the ideal bond between the bone and the component will be achieved.

If an uncemented acetabular component is to be used, then keyholes are not made. However, the acetabular cavity is reamed to a known size, often 50 to 52 mm (about 2 in) in diameter. The acetabular metal backing is then taken and hammered in place. It is normal to ream the acetabulum to a size 1 or 2 mm (under ⅟₁₆ in) smaller than the component finally chosen. This is referred to as *press-fit*. It ensures that the acetabular component is well fixed into the surrounding bone. Screws may also be used to fix the acetabulum in place.

The surgical team then turns its attention to the femur. Cylindrical reamers are now used to ream a channel down the middle of the femoral shaft. A decision will again have been taken before the operation as to whether a cemented or cementless femoral component is to be used. For a cemented design, once the femoral canal has been reamed, it is usual to place a *cement restrictor* down the middle of the femoral canal. This is to ensure that any cement inserted does not disappear to the very end of the femur. Cement is only needed in the region of the femoral component and as little as possible should be inserted to achieve the desired effect.

Once the femoral canal has been reamed, it is cleaned and dried. The cement is then inserted, pressurized and then the femoral component is inserted at the last moment. The surgeon holds the component in position and keeps it completely still until the cement has set. If a cementless femoral component is used, then under-reaming, as mentioned above, ensures a good press-fit.

If a modular design is being used, the ball is applied to the femoral component at this point, the two new parts of the hip then being pressed back together to form the new joint. Balls come in various sizes, and also in various lengths. It is the *length* of the ball that is important at this stage if the surgeon is to ensure that the legs are as much the same length as each other as possible. Getting them exactly the same length is a difficult thing to achieve at hip surgery, but a modular design gives the surgeon a good chance of doing so.

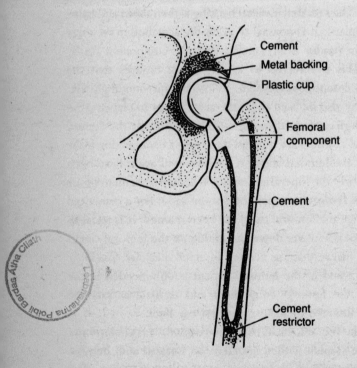

Cement
Metal backing
Plastic cup

Femoral
component

Cement

Cement
restrictor

Figure 6.2 *A primary total hip replacement. A cemented, metal-backed acetabular component has been used, with a cemented femoral component.*

If a cemented hip replacement is used (see Figure 6.2), an antibiotic may be mixed into the cement. The commonest antibiotic used in bone cement is called gentamicin. This provides high levels of antibiotic action in the immediate area of the hip replacement, further aiding the efforts made to reduce the chance of infection.

Once the replacement hip has been inserted, its stability is assessed. The surgeon sees if the ball will remain in the socket or pop out of joint with little effort, that is, *dislocate*. Dislocation can be a major handicap to a patient and it is important that the surgeon leaves the hip joint as stable as possible at the end of the operation. If there is evidence of instability, there are a number of things the surgeon can do to minimize the problem.

An assessment can also be made as to whether or not particular movements are likely to prove troublesome once the patient wakes up. Post-operatively advice can then be given for the patient to avoid such movements until full healing has occurred.

Once stability has been assessed and is seen to be satisfactory, the incision is then closed. Small plastic tubes (*drains*) may be inserted in order to remove any blood that oozes after the operation. Some surgeons do not use drains, though, as they believe they may pose a risk of infection.

AFTER THE OPERATION

Once the final skin stitch, or staple, has been inserted, the patient is transferred from the operating table to bed. It is usual at this stage for the leg to be held in some form of immobilizing device. The simplest and most widely used of these is an *abduction pillow*. This is a triangular pillow that is placed between the patient's legs to hold them apart. This abducted position is the most stable position that a hip can adopt and so it is the safest position in which a patient can lie in the early post-operative phase. It reduces the chances of dislocation occurring after the operation before the patient is fully awake. However, not all surgeons use an abduction pillow at this stage.

Once transferred to a bed, the patient is taken to the recovery room. Though the anaesthetist will have removed the breathing tube in the operating theatre, it may take several minutes before the patient will have woken sufficiently to be able to breathe and swallow safely and independently. It is therefore the task of recovery room staff to ensure that this gradual reawakening occurs in safe and supervised surroundings. The recovery room is equipped with emergency equipment should problems occur at this stage. An anaesthetist may also be on hand for maximum safety.

Once the patient has fully recovered consciousness, they are returned to the ward. For a routine hip replacement operation, though the surgical operating time is only 80 minutes, the total time away from the ward can be as much as 3 hours. This time includes the giving of anaesthetic, its taking effect, surgery and waking up from the anaesthetic. Relatives who are awaiting news of their loved ones and how they are doing, often become alarmed at the length of time the operation appears to take. So, it is important that they are made aware of all that is involved in the operation so that they know that a three-hour absence from the ward does not mean that there are problems.

7

COMPLICATIONS OF HIP REPLACEMENT OPERATIONS

The aim of this chapter is not to depress you but to make sure that you are aware of possible outcomes of total hip replacement surgery. What is important is that someone does not end up in a worse condition than they experienced prior to their operation. You can only make a responsible decision about whether or not to proceed with a hip replacement when you have a full picture of what is involved.

Complications are many and varied. Most are minor, associated with surgery in general rather than being specific to hip replacement. Only the minority of complications are to the long-term detriment of the patient. However, for the older patient, the chances of complications occurring increase. For patients over the age of 80, for example, it has been shown that 20 per cent of them will experience some form of post-operative complication. Revision hip surgery is also associated with a higher rate of complications than are primary replacements.

Throughout this chapter an idea of the likely level of risk is given for each complication, expressed in percentage terms. The figures are those given in scientific papers published in the major orthopaedic journals, but note figures given by different pieces of research often vary widely, so any figures provided can only be a rough guide. Sometimes it has not been possible to give an accurate estimate of the risk, in which case no figure has been quoted.

Complications may be grouped into three main categories:

1 operative
2 post-operative
3 long-term (six months or more after surgery).

These three categories will be considered in turn.

Operative Complications

This group of complications encompasses those that take place while surgery is in progress. They may be classified as follows:

- neurological
- vascular
- cortical perforation
- fracture
- legs of unequal length
- entrapped drain
- cement extrusion
- to do with the anaesthetic.

NEUROLOGICAL COMPLICATIONS (RISK: 0.5–3.5 PER CENT)

In the immediate vicinity of the hip joint are a number of nerves that are important for controlling the lower limb normally. A nerve may be cut accidentally, retracted by the assistant too brusquely or stretched if a limb is made longer as part of the operation. For example, a patient may develop osteoarthritis of the hip joint as the result of a long-standing congenital dislocation of the hip. In order to replace the joint it is sometimes necessary to lengthen the leg significantly. This lengthening can stretch the nerves around the hip joint and cause them to malfunction. Lengthening a leg more than 4 cm (1½ in) significantly increases the chances of nerve damage being caused. The leg should therefore be lengthened as little as possible.

Scientific studies on the functioning of nerves after hip replacement show that more than 15 per cent of patients show some evidence of mild damage. In one study, 21 out of 30 patients showed evidence of damage. Fortunately, the majority of patients recover, unaware of any problem at all. In a very small percentage of patients – less than 0.5 per cent – nerve damage can be a permanent feature.

VASCULAR COMPLICATIONS (RISK: LESS THAN 0.1 PER CENT FOR PRIMARY REPLACEMENTS; LESS THAN 1 PER CENT FOR REVISION REPLACEMENTS)

Running alongside most nerves may be found blood vessels. In any operation there are a number of blind spots where the surgeon knows there is likely to be a problem, but is unable to physically see it. A good example is the femoral artery. This lies immediately to the front of the acetabulum and can sometimes be damaged during surgery. The femoral vein lies in the same area and can also be damaged. If it is, the surgeon may need to make further incisions or to lengthen the original incision in order to control the bleeding. Only rarely does vascular damage threaten the leg itself.

CORTICAL PERFORATION (RISK: UP TO 4.5 PER CENT)

At the time of surgery, every attempt is made to ensure that all instruments passed down the femoral canal do go down the very middle of it. In practice, though, this is sometimes difficult, particularly in revision operations. On such occasions it is possible that the surgeon, when reaming, will breach the side of the femur, making a cortical perforation (see Figure 7.1). The *cortex* of the femur is the hard, outer part of the bone. The *medulla* is the spongy, inner area.

A cortical perforation does not usually cause great problems for the patient. Indeed, the majority of patients would be unaware of it if one occurred. The surgeon may choose to leave the perforation as it is, to bone graft the defect, to fill it with cement or to use a femoral component that has a longer stem to bypass and strengthen the now weakened area.

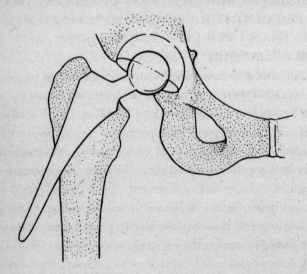

Figure 7.1 *Cortical perforation. This looks bad, but patients are frequently unaware it has happened!*

FRACTURE (RISK: LESS THAN 1 PER CENT FOR PRIMARY REPLACEMENTS; APPROXIMATELY 3 PER CENT FOR REVISION REPLACEMENTS)

It is sometimes possible for the surgeon to fracture the patient's bone during the operation. This is most likely during either revision surgery, when the patient's own bone has deteriorated, or when a cementless femoral component is being inserted. Many of the cementless components rely for their success on a very tight press-fit. The process of reaming the bone or inserting the component can therefore cause fractures.

In the majority of cases, such fractures are not a problem. They are usually tiny, hairline cracks that mend in time. In the minority of cases, a fracture can be a major problem and additional techniques will need to be used to fix the new joint in place during surgery. Sometimes, the surgeon will elect to leave the fracture as it is and treat the patient in bed for several weeks after the procedure.

LEGS OF UNEQUAL LENGTH (RISK OF DIFFERENCE OF MORE THAN 1 CM (⅜ IN), 6 PER CENT FOR PRIMARY REPLACEMENTS; 7.5 PER CENT FOR REVISION REPLACEMENTS)

To non-surgeons it must seem odd that surgery to the hip joint can result in the legs becoming unequal in length. However, to obtain a precise length match is, in fact, sometimes very difficult.

If an error *is* made, it is more usual to overlengthen the operated on side than to shorten it. Functionally, it rarely poses problems, unless the overlengthening is associated with nerve damage (see under Neurological complications above). Cosmetically, though, it is obviously of concern to the patient, particularly as it may be necessary to wear a raised shoe on the unoperated on side in order to keep the hip level.

For revision surgery, the failed primary replacement is often associated with shortening of that leg. Patients will naturally ask whether or not it is possible to regain the lost length. This is difficult and assurances are hard to give. Sometimes the surgeon actually has to lengthen the leg in order to ensure stability of the hip replacement, but, if it is a choice between a dislocating hip replacement and an increase in leg length, most surgeons will choose increased leg length for the patient's sake.

ENTRAPPED DRAIN

Drains are frequently left in the incision for a 48-hour period in order to ensure thorough removal of any post-operative bleeding. Occasionally, they can inadvertently be sutured into the deeper areas of the incision. This makes it impossible to remove them without a further operation.

Should such a thing happen, the drain could theoretically be left safely where it lay, deep inside the patient. It is unlikely, and of course understandable, that a patient will accept this and, thus, a further operation to remove it may be required.

CEMENT EXTRUSION

During cementation of a cemented hip replacement, great pressure is applied to the cement to ensure it spreads into every little crevice of the bone. Sometimes the pressure applied causes the cement to push through (extrude) the inner wall of the acetabulum or around its margins. Sometimes it can be pushed through a small hole in the cortex of the femur.

In practice this is not a problem, though there are a few reports that cement extrusion has caused damage to vital structures. However, in the majority of cases, cement extrusion causes no problems and merely shows up as an odd shape on an X-ray. Most pieces of extruded cement should be left where they are.

COMPLICATIONS WITH THE ANAESTHETIC

Complications arising regarding the anaesthetic cannot be covered in full detail here as anaesthesia is a vast topic, but the following is a summary of the most important points to be borne in mind.

Many complications can be avoided by carefully assessing patients prior to surgery, screening out those with certain conditions that put them at risk of complications and taking steps to settle such problems pre-operatively if surgery is unavoidable, while others can be minimized by taking special precautions with the anaesthetic during surgery. The conditions that greatly increase the risk of complications include:

- high blood pressure (*hypertension*)
- severe heart disease (there is a 35 per cent chance of death after surgery if a patient has had a heart attack within the previous 3 months)
- respiratory disease
- chronic kidney disease
- certain hormonal diseases, such as diabetes
- assorted, miscellaneous problems, such as severe cases of rheumatoid arthritis and stiff necks and reduced jaw mobility as this makes it difficult to insert the tubes needed for artificial respiration.

Hip replacement may be performed under general or local anaesthetic, both of which may be associated with complications. Such problems are not confined to orthopaedic surgery alone, but to surgery in general. Occasionally, both local and general anaesthetic can be administered at the same operation.

A significant part of an anaesthetist's role is to ensure that the patient does not lose too much blood during the operation. Any blood lost can be replaced throughout the operation by the anaesthetist. However, sometimes the patient reacts abnormally to the transfused blood – called a *transfusion reaction*.

To minimize blood loss and thus the need for transfusion and the possibility of a transfusion reaction, the technique of *hypotensive anaesthesia* is sometimes used. This is when the patient's blood pressure is intentionally lowered (*hypotension*) in order to reduce bleeding. The use of local anaesthesia can reduce blood loss still further. The drawback of this technique is that unusually pronounced, or prolonged, hypotensive anaesthesia can damage the kidneys, heart and brain. Its use should therefore be confined to those who are experienced in the technique and it should be used for short periods only.

When the cement is inserted, it is possible for some of the cement liquid (known as *monomer*) to escape into the bloodstream and be circulated round the body. Also, small globules of fat can enter the bloodstream when the bone is being prepared – a situation known as *fat embolism*. In either case, the blood pressure can drop dramatically and, in some cases, lead to a patient dying on the operating table. For this reason, the surgeon usually warns the anaesthetist before inserting cement into the patient. Then the anaesthetist can be prepared to counteract sudden falls in the blood pressure if they should occur.

When a patient is anaesthetized, it is difficult for the body to keep warm, particularly where special air flow systems are used in operating theatres. This exposes the patient to the risk of a reduced body temperature, known as *hypothermia*. This is a particular risk in the elderly.

Post-operative Complications

These are diverse but may be grouped under the following headings:

* neurological
* dislocation
* infection
* trochanteric problems
* gastrointestinal complications
* urinary complications
* cardiovascular complications
* miscellaneous complications.

NEUROLOGICAL COMPLICATIONS

The majority of neurological complications occur at the time of the operation. However, if blood continues to leak out *after* the operation, it can collect around one or other of the major nerves in the vicinity of the hip joint. This can cause a delayed nerve palsy. This, though, occurs rarely.

DISLOCATION (RISK: 0.5–3 PER CENT)

When the ball of the hip replacement becomes disconnected from the socket of the acetabulum, this is *dislocation* (see Figure 7.2). It can sometimes occur because of where the various components have been inserted or because of poor muscle tone in the area of the joint replacement. Some surgical approaches are said to be associated with higher dislocation rates than others, but, in practice, this is probably not a cause. Surgeons may notice that their dislocation rate reduces as they gain more experience using a particular approach, irrespective of *which* approach they use.

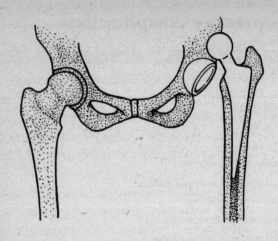

Figure 7.2 *Dislocation. The risk of dislocation exists for life, particularly when the hip joint is bent to more than 90 degrees.*

If the hip dislocates, it is likely that it will only happen once. The hip will then be reduced, and that will be an end to it. For the minority of patients, though, dislocation will continue to be a problem and they will become a *recurrent dislocator*. In such cases, special surgical appliances may have to be worn or a revision operation may be needed. Revision surgery to correct recurrent dislocation is difficult and so many patients who have this problem continue to be recurrent dislocators, despite the best efforts of the revision hip surgeon.

INFECTION (RISK: 7 PER CENT FOR SUPERFICIAL INFECTION; 0.5 PER CENT FOR DEEP INFECTION)

The incidence of infection following total hip replacement is variable. Infection may be *superficial* or *deep*. Superficial infection is when the infection is confined to the superficial tissues only – the skin and immediately subcutaneous structures. The site of the incision appears hot and red, but this soon responds to antibiotics.

Deep infection is different. Here the infection involves the hip replacement itself and this is harder to eradicate. Also, superficial infections can *become* deep infections if they are left untreated. This is why orthopaedic surgeons take any form of infection very seriously. Indeed, some surgeons believe there is no such thing as a superficial infection, treating *any* infection as deep infection.

Every effort is made to reduce the chances of infection occurring – giving antibiotic treatment, using special air flow systems within the operating theatre and sterile techniques. Despite all these precautions, infection can occur. When it does, revision surgery is often required and, although it is likely to solve the problem, it cannot always be *guaranteed* to do so. Revision surgery itself is associated with a higher rate of infection than primary hip replacement.

TROCHANTERIC PROBLEMS (RISK: 9.5 PER CENT FOR TROCHANTERIC NON-UNION; UP TO 17 PER CENT FOR TROCHANTERIC BURSITIS)

Certain surgical techniques require the removal of the greater trochanter, at the upper end of the femur. The trochanter is then re-attached at the end of the operation. Re-attachment is important because the hip abductor muscles are attached to the trochanter. Occasionally, the greater trochanter fails to heal back in place, despite the wires that are often used to secure it. This is called a *non-union*. Should this happen, then the greater trochanter can pull off in an upwards direction and, though not a serious complication, it may be necessary to re-attach it in another operation.

Even if a trochanter does heal back into position, the

patient may still experience pain on the outer part of the hip following surgery. This is sometimes called *trochanteric bursitis* and may occasionally require further surgery. The risk of developing trochanteric bursitis post-operatively exists even if the greater trochanter is *not* removed during the operation. However, the chances of it happening are much less.

GASTROINTESTINAL COMPLICATIONS (RISK: SLIGHTLY MORE THAN 1 PER CENT)

The hip joint is separated from part of the gastrointestinal tract by a thin shell of bone on the inner part of the acetabulum. As a result, it is possible for the bowels to take time to recover after surgery. Sometimes they are totally inactive for a while – a phenomenon known as *ileus*. This usually resolves itself spontaneously, though sometimes an intravenous infusion, combined with a temporary tube swallowed into the stomach, is required to get them working normally again.

Occasionally, particularly in the elderly, it is possible for the tract to become infected. This may happen when antibiotic therapy is given. The antibiotics used to prevent the hip replacement being infected can sometimes suppress the normal bacteria within the gastrointestinal tract. This allows abnormal bacteria to flourish, gastroenteritis being the result. Occasionally a period of barrier nursing will be required while the tract recovers.

URINARY COMPLICATIONS (RISK: UP TO 35 PER CENT)

As the hip joint is near to the soft tissue structures of the pelvis, it is possible for the urinary system to stop functioning normally after the operation. This is particularly common in men, whose prostate glands may be enlarged and who can sometimes find it very difficult to pass urine post-operatively.

When urine cannot be passed at all, the situation is known as *urinary retention*. It is sometimes necessary for a tube to be passed up the penis and into the bladder, the tube being known as a *urinary catheter*. Occasionally, it is necessary for men to undergo removal of the prostate gland soon after hip replacement surgery as a result of urinary problems. This occurs in 0.25 per cent of cases.

Urinary retention can also occur in women. In such cases, it is usually because it is difficult to pass urine while lying in bed. Again, a urinary catheter inserted for a while after surgery can help. Surgeons like to avoid inserting urinary catheters if possible as they pose a risk of infection. However, this risk is sometimes unavoidable.

Urinary tract infection can sometimes occur after hip replacement (risk: 4.5 per cent). This is sometimes because an infection was not diagnosed pre-operatively or because the patient develops it as a result of poor urine flow post-operatively. This is usually treated with antibiotics as soon as it is diagnosed.

CARDIOVASCULAR COMPLICATIONS (RISK: UP TO 56 PER CENT)

Cardiovascular complications are problems associated with the heart and blood vessels.

The stress of surgery is sometimes so great for those with weak hearts that a heart attack (*myocardial infarction* – risk: less than 0.5 per cent) can occur. This is a serious situation, but only very rarely results in death.

Occasionally a blood clot can form in the brain – a stroke (*cerebrovascular accident*). This is rare and usually mild and recovery is normally complete, but, unfortunately, it does not always occur.

The commonest cardiovascular complication is the *deep vein thrombosis* (DVT), which is when blood clots form in the deep veins of the legs (the veins deep inside the calf and thigh that cannot be seen from the surface). The reasons for DVT occurring in patients who have undergone surgery have been argued for years, but a clear explanation is still awaited. The condition is commoner in women than men. If preventative treatment is not provided, then 35 per cent of patients under the age of 60 years will develop a DVT, and 56 per cent of those over 70 will do so.

A small percentage of patients with a DVT can demonstrate the potentially life-threatening condition of a *pulmonary embolism*. This occurs when a small piece of blood clot breaks free and passes into the general circulation of the blood, passes through the heart and stops in the lungs. The majority of pulmonary emboli are minor and can be easily treated. The minority can result in death. Up to 3.6 per cent of patients undergoing a hip replacement will experience a pulmonary embolism.

The commonest time for DVTs to appear and for pulmonary emboli to occur is approximately ten days after surgery, though the risk of an embolism is still present four weeks after surgery. This is a complication that orthopaedic surgeons take very seriously.

MISCELLANEOUS COMPLICATIONS

Haematoma Formation (risk: 3 per cent)

A *haematoma* is a collection of blood deep under the skin. Sometimes it is possible for one of the drains to block, thereby allowing blood to collect within the patient, rather than in the drain bottle. Normally, this is not a problem. Occasionally, there is such a large haematoma that it can discharge via the incision. The blood of a haematoma is dark red and thick. Even though it is not usually a problem medically, it can be distressing for the patient.

Wound Dehiscence

A *dehiscence* of a wound is when part or all of the incision fails to heal. In very elderly people or those who are taking steroids (for example, patients with rheumatoid arthritis), it is possible that the incision will not heal in the expected time. When sutures are removed, small areas of the incision can gape or, occasionally, the whole of it can split open from top to bottom. Should this happen, further suturing of the incision is required.

This is an uncommon complication, the risk of an incision having to be reopened and resutured after a hip replacement operation being 0.05 per cent for both primary and revision operations.

Respiratory Complications (risk: slightly less than 1 per cent)

Due to the length of the operation and the time the patient is under general anaesthetic, the amount of air getting to parts of the lungs may be reduced. This can cause infection within the respiratory tract, usually within two to three days of surgery. Treatment involves physiotherapy, antibiotics and ensuring that the patient is mobile as soon as possible. The more active the patient is, the better is the flow of air through the lungs and the less trouble respiratory infection is likely to create for them.

Prosthetic Displacement

Rarely, the femoral or acetabular components shift in position soon after the operation. This is despite the best efforts of the surgeon to fix them in place as securely as possible. More frequently with the cementless designs, that often rely on a good press-fit being achieved, than the cemented ones, it is almost unknown for this to occur while the patient is in hospital. Usually, if it is going to happen, displacement occurs within the first six months after surgery and so it is considered a post-operative complication.

Should either component shift in position, it is unlikely that the surgeon will do much beyond observing the situation. If component shift becomes a danger to the patient or their mobility, then further surgery may be required.

Knee Pain

Patients sometimes complain of pain and swelling in the knee of the operated on leg after surgery. This may be due to associated arthritis, the knee also being a weight-bearing joint. However, it can also be due to the twisting and turning of the leg that is required during surgery. Sometimes it can take the knee joint several weeks to recover. It is not a serious complication and usually fully settles.

Swollen Ankle or Ankles

Patients commonly complain of a swollen ankle or ankles after surgery. This may be related to the presence of a deep vein thrombosis (DVT), but may also be due to limited mobility. In the normal, fully active person, the body has a *muscle pump* that helps drive blood back to the heart. After a hip replacement operation, a patient is confined to bed for several days. This can result in swelling of the ankle or ankles. This usually subsides completely within three months of surgery and is not a significant complication.

Skin Complications (risk: less than 1 per cent)

After the incision is stitched, it is possible for the skin edges to die. This is known as *skin necrosis*. It is not a serious complication, but skin healing may be delayed should it occur.

Pressure sores (sometimes called *bed sores* or *decubitus ulceration*) are more significant. Usually seen in the elderly, they are often to be found on the heels and bottom. Occasionally, they may be found over the greater trochanter of the opposite, unoperated on, hip due to the length of time spent in one position on the operating table. Such sores are caused by prolonged periods of pressure on the skin. They can normally be avoided by carefully assessing the patient on admission and by giving precise, attentive nursing care. If a pressure sore should occur, it can take many months to settle and may occasionally require a skin grafting operation to clear it up.

Metabolic Complications (risk: less than 1 per cent)

Disorders of the body's metabolism are infrequent. Rarely, the kidneys can cease to function (*renal failure*). A more common metabolic problem is the development of gout, a build-up of a substance called *uric acid* in the blood. This is easily treated with medicines.

Death (risk: approximately 1 per cent)

Deaths related to hip replacement operations are rare, but, as with all operations, it should be recognized as a risk.

Long-term Complications

Long-term complications are problems that occur six months or more after a hip replacement operation. They are as follows:

- aseptic loosening
- bone stock loss
- component fracture
- late dislocation
- late infection
- bone fracture
- ectopic ossification.

ASEPTIC LOOSENING

Aseptic loosening occurs when components become loose but not because of the presence of an infection. It is usually caused by wear particles produced as a result of friction in the artificial hip (see page 53). These wear particles set up a low-grade inflammatory reaction that eventually results in loss of the patient's own bone, a phenomenon known as *osteolysis*. This is the commonest cause of long-term failure of a total hip replacement.

One way in which aseptic loosening can be identified as early as possible is by taking regular X-rays. This is why some surgeons ask to see their patients for follow-up appointments on a regular basis after surgery. Evidence of loosening can be seen in X-ray photographs in approximately 4.5 per cent of patients a year after surgery, and 30 per cent after 10 years. This figure can be as high as 40 per cent after 10 years for certain designs of component.

BONE STOCK LOSS

As a primary hip replacement begins to loosen — whether this be due to infection or aseptic loosening — it is possible for the patient's own bone to slowly disappear. This is a problem that is addressed in revision surgery, usually by using bone grafting techniques.

COMPONENT FRACTURE (RISK: UP TO 11 PER CENT FOR THE FEMORAL COMPONENT IN CERTAIN STUDIES, THOUGH FIGURES ARE LARGELY FROM THE MID 1970S)

As with any man-made material, fatigue can be a problem. This can occasionally result in the fracture of either a femoral or, more rarely, an acetabular component. The ceramic ball used as a femoral head can also fracture (risk: 7 per cent between 2 weeks and 27 months post-operatively).

Component fracture is now a rare complication, but was common in the 1970s and 1980s before many components were strengthened. A broken femoral component can cause great technical troubles in revision surgery. Special equipment has been designed to enable surgeons to cope with this situation if it arises. A fractured acetabular component is very rare, usually affecting the thinner-walled designs if it occurs.

LATE DISLOCATION (RISK: 2 PER CENT)

A late dislocation can occur even in a hip replacement that has no previous history of instability. By definition, a late dislocation is one that occurs six years or more after the original operation. This probably happens because of increased muscle weakness as a patient gets older, combined with stretching of the tissues that surround the replacement hip. It can prove a difficult problem to solve and may require a revision operation.

LATE INFECTION (RISK: LESS THAN 1 PER CENT)

It is possible for a hip replacement to become infected many years after the initial operation. Sometimes it can happen because other surgical procedures release bacteria into the bloodstream, some of which lodge in the hip replacement. Dental procedures are occasionally blamed and sometimes urinary tract procedures. For this reason, any hip replacement patient who subsequently undergoes some other form of surgery, whatever it may be, should inform the relevant medical staff that they have a hip replacement.

BONE FRACTURE (RISK: SLIGHTLY LESS THAN 1 PER CENT)

Because of the reduction in the patient's own bone strength due to aseptic loosening, it is possible for either the femur or acetabulum to become very weak and thin. This weakness can become so great that a fracture occurs. If the femur fractures, it normally happens near the tip of the femoral component. This can pose an enormous challenge to the revision hip surgeon. Such fractures can heal naturally, though surgery is often required.

ECTOPIC OSSIFICATION (RISK: 7 PER CENT FOR PRIMARY REPLACEMENT; 15 PER CENT FOR REVISION REPLACEMENT)

Ectopic ossification, sometimes known as *heterotopic ossification*, is the formation of bone in the soft tissues that surround the hip. It usually takes the form of small islands of bone that cause no problems to the patient, but show up as strange shapes on an X-ray. However, ectopic bone can sometimes spread extensively. In the worst case, it can grow to fill the space between femur and acetabulum, preventing all hip joint movement (see Figure 7.3). It is very difficult to rectify once established.

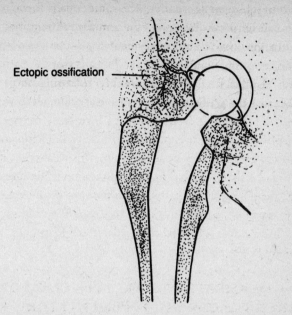

Ectopic ossification

Figure 7.3 *Ectopic ossification. Sometimes known as heterotopic ossification, it can occasionally be very severe and prevent all movement of the new hip joint.*

Salvage Procedures

Occasionally, complications associated with a total hip replacement are such that it is not possible to correct the situation with reconstructive surgery without exposing the patient to undue risk. In such a situation, operations known as *salvage procedures* are applied.

Excision arthroplasty (see pages 18 – 19) is one such salvage procedure. Surgeons have occasionally attempted to fuse (*arthrodesis*) the hip joint once a hip replacement has failed. However, this is technically difficult because of the poor quality of bone associated with the previous hip replacement.

Amputation is also an alternative when there really is nothing else that can be done. However, the amputation required in such a situation – known as a *hindquarter amputation* – is a large operation, no simple undertaking, and means that the patient will have significantly reduced mobility following surgery. This is because the artificial limbs available are difficult to wear and use.

8

REVISION HIP REPLACEMENT – THE OPERATION

Revision hip replacement is an expanding part of modern orthopaedic surgery. However well a primary hip replacement performs, and for however long, it is possible that it will one day fail. When a primary hip replacement is re-performed, it is referred to as a *revision*.

In the early days of hip replacement, revision operations were regarded by many as ones to be avoided. Because the operation was difficult to perform and results were then likely to be bad, little thought was given as to how things might be improved. As primary hip replacements became more common, though, the number of revision operations necessary rose and so there was a need to develop the techniques of revision surgery to a more advanced level.

There were a few early pioneers, but recent years have shown orthopaedic specialists being appointed to new posts specifically to perform revision surgery. Courses are now run worldwide to teach surgeons the exacting techniques involved and the development of instruments used has proceeded apace. Revision hip surgery has earned itself a respected place within the specialism of orthopaedics and its results have significantly improved.

Much of the care of the patient before, during and after the operation is identical to that associated with a primary hip replacement (see Chapter 6). However, there are aspects of revision hip surgery that are specific to it and these are now discussed.

Pre-operative Assessment

As with a primary hip replacement, a revision patient may need to be assessed ahead of time to ensure that blood is cross-matched, any urinary tract infections are treated and an over-all assessment is made as to whether or not they are well enough to undergo surgery. In a revision operation, blood loss is likely to be greater and so more blood will need to be made available than is customary for a primary replacement.

One important assessment that needs to be made by the orthopaedic surgeon is whether or not the primary hip replacement is infected. This is something that should prefer-ably be known before a revision operation is undertaken. If revision hip surgery takes place when an undiagnosed infection exists, it is possible that the revision replacement will fail because the infection could simply recur. However, it is some-times very difficult to know whether or not a hip replacement is infected. Orthopaedic infections rarely appear as abscesses or the patient feeling unwell, but, rather, they can appear as little more than minor discomfort. If an infection has been present in a primary hip replacement for many years, it can also be a cause of loosening. To assist the surgeon in making a diagnosis of infection, a number of blood tests, scans and a procedure known as *aspiration* can be used.

The two most common blood tests performed in this situa-tion are the *erythrocyte sedimentation rate* (ESR) and *C-reactive protein* (CRP). When these tests produce an abnormal result, this suggests that an infection is present. Such results would not be conclusive proof of an infection but are a useful indicator.

More specific indicators are *isotope scans*. X-rays are difficult to interpret in such situations, particularly in the early post-operative days. Isotope scans provide more information. These involve the injection of a radio-isotope into the patient and the uptake of that radio-isotope being measured at various points in the body. The commonest radio-isotopes used are *technetium*, *gallium* or *indium*. The technetium scan is a broad indicator as to whether or not a hip replacement is loose, while the gallium and indium scans are more specifically for showing the prescence, or absence, of infection.

Finally, an aspiration may be performed. This is a minor operation performed under local or general anaesthetic and involves passing a needle into the hip replacement to remove fluid from it. The fluid is sent to a bacteriology laboratory as soon as it has been extracted. It is the most accurate way to establish what is happening within a hip replacement.

With such tests available, it is usually possible for the orthopaedic surgeon to have a good idea as to whether or not the hip replacement is infected before a revision operation is undertaken and, thus, the operation can be planned reasonably accurately. It would be wrong to claim that infections can *always* be diagnosed as sometimes the tests do not pick it up and it only becomes obvious during the operation.

If *no* infection is present, the orthopaedic surgeon is likely to suggest a *one-stage* revision operation. This is the removal of the primary hip replacement and the insertion of a new hip replacement, all in one operation. However, if infection is present, the surgeon may recommend a *two-stage* revision operation.

The first of the two stages is the removal of the primary hip replacement, leaving the patient without a hip joint for a time.

This is referred to as an *excision arthroplasty*, similar to the Girdlestone procedure described on pages 18 – 19.

The patient will commonly remain with an excision arthroplasty for six weeks, but periods up to one year are sometimes known. The length of time is determined by the nature of the bacteria causing the infection: the stronger the bacteria, the longer the patient must remain with an excision arthroplasty. The patient does not always have to stay in hospital between the first and second stages. The absence of a hip joint does not mean walking is impossible. It is unlikely that the patient would be able to walk without support, but it should still be possible to get about without help.

Once the infection has settled, the second-stage operation is performed and a revision hip replacement is inserted. After this, mobility can be as good as that following primary hip replacement, though the degree of mobility is harder to predict.

The Operation

A patient going into hospital for a revision operation will be prepared for it in a similar way to a patient receiving a primary replacement. The only difference is that it is less likely that the operation will take place under local anaesthetic because it takes much longer (generally up to three to four hours, sometimes more).

During surgery, the surgeons may have to modify their usual approach. It may be, for example, that a posterior approach would normally be used for a primary operation whereas in a revision operation, a number of other specialist techniques would need to be used to retrieve the various components of the failed hip safely. Sometimes the operation needs to take place on the inside of the pelvis, rather than on the outside. This happens when the acetabular cup has failed and has shifted inwards towards the bladder and other soft tissue organs in the pelvis.

Using such techniques, the surgeon must first remove the primary hip replacement. This is not always easy. The replacement may have been in place for more than a decade, a cement restrictor may not have been used in the femur and the acetabular component may have shifted markedly. In the early days of revision surgery, there was no specialized equipment to help the surgeon cope with these circumstances. This is no longer the case and so the results of the revision operations have improved. Cement is extremely hard and it is very difficult to remove from the very depths of a thin femoral canal without damaging the femur itself. *High-speed cutting drills* may be used that have centralizing devices to ensure that drill holes are made down the very *middle* of the bone, not through the side. Lasers have occasionally been recommended and *ultrasound* can also be used. However, for the majority of cases, it is possible to remove the old components and cement using hand-held instruments called *cementotomes*. These are hardened metal, chisel-like instruments that split cement easily. However, the surgeon must take care to split only the cement, not the surrounding bone.

Once the old hip replacement, including any cement, has been removed, the revision hip components can be inserted. This process is referred to as *reconstruction* and the components may be either cemented or cementless. Revision hip surgeons fall into two groups. There are those who believe in cemented reconstruction and those who believe in cementless techniques. The cemented reconstructors argue that sufficiently good results cannot be achieved with cementless components. The cementless reconstructors argue that fixing the revision hip in place with cement can compound the situation that has already been caused by a cemented component being inserted in the first place. Perhaps the truth lies somewhere between these two extremes. There are some patients for whom a cemented revision is more suitable than a cementless one and vice versa. It is an individual decision.

Frequently, because a primary hip replacement has been in place for a number of years, the patient's own bone will have begun to disappear. This is referred to as loss of bone stock (see page 12). Most revision surgeons would agree that to insert a revision replacement against weak bone is to invite it to fail prematurely. Great efforts are therefore made to reconstruct the bone stock before the revision components are inserted.

The bone can be rebuilt by using either the patient's own bone (*autograft*) or another person's bone (*allograft*). When autograft bone is used, this is normally removed from the patient's own pelvis. Because the pelvis has had a hip replacement in place for some years, it is unlikely that there will be sufficient autograft bone available for reconstruction. It is more likely therefore, that the orthopaedic surgeon will use allograft bone.

Allograft bone comes from bone banks. These are cold storage units in which donated bone has been kept. The bone may have been donated at the time of a primary replacement when the femoral head was removed or it may come from multiorgan donors, who donate organs for transplantation, such as kidneys and heart, as well as bone. Bone banks regularly supply orthopaedic departments in the countries in which they exist with allograft bone for revision hip surgery. Not all countries run a bone banking system as there are sometimes religious, political and financial objections to their existence, but, where they do exist, they make a significant contribution to the success of revision hip surgery.

If autograft or allograft bone is not available, surgeons may consider the use of either *bone substitutes* or *xenograft*. Bone substitutes are materials that are manufactured specifically to replace bone. Their use is not currently widespread. Xenograft is bone from animals. Again, this is not widely used as results are sometimes unpredictable.

In revision surgery, once the depleted bone has been reconstructed, the surgeon must then insert the revision hip components. Often it is possible to use components that are designed for primary hip replacement, though this is not always the case. Special femoral components do exist, some with longer stems, some with broader bodies and some that are specially reinforced, in order to cater for the wide variety of situations that present themselves in revision hip surgery. For the acetabular component, to prevent a recurrence of the shifting inwards that happens (a phenomenon known as *protrusio*), special reinforcement rings exist. These are metal rings that attach to the outer wall of the pelvis, usually with hooks and screws, to fill the defect in the patient's own bone.

Post-operative Care

Once the operation is over, the post-operative care the patient will receive is similar to that received following primary hip replacement (see pages 73 – 4). However, it may be necessary to use crutches for longer and for a special hip brace to be worn for a time. The brace keeps the new hip replacement in a safe position until the soft tissues have repaired.

The stay in hospital is normally the same as for primary hip replacement, though a stay of up to half as long again can be expected when surgery is more complicated. If infection has been a problem, then it may also be necessary for antibiotics to be given for longer periods than would otherwise be the case.

9

THE RESULTS OF HIP REPLACEMENT OPERATIONS

'How long will it last, doctor?' is a question that many patients will ask their orthopaedic surgeon prior to a hip replacement operation. To give an accurate reply is impossible, but most orthopaedic surgeons will advise that an average of ten years is a realistic estimate. It should be remembered that this is an *average* and *not* a guarantee. A total hip replacement is a man-made device. Surgery involves putting this device in contact with living, natural bone. The body treats the hip replacement as a large foreign body, similar to a splinter. It tries to wall it off from the rest of the body, surrounding it with a thick membrane. The materials now used for total hip replacement components cause sufficiently low amounts of irritation as to ensure that most patients do not react to them. Rarely, an allergic response can occur.

Irrespective of the *type* of replacement performed, more than 95 per cent of patients are highly satisfied with the results of surgery in the immediate post-operative period. As time goes by, the components begin to loosen (see Figure 9.1) and so the level of satisfaction declines. For an operation that is so widely and frequently performed, there are few long-term follow-up studies of total hip replacements. Certain centres

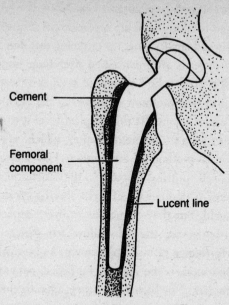

Cement

Femoral
component

Lucent line

Figure 9.1 *Aseptic loosening of a hip replacement. Note the gap which has appeared around the cemented femoral component. This is sometimes called a lucent line.*

dominate the research field in the accuracy of the data they collect.

The problem of following up total hip replacement patients after surgery is partly created by the success of the operation itself. If a surgeon performs 100 hip replacements per year, then, in a 10-year period, 1000 replacements will have been performed by that surgeon. Each patient should, ideally, be seen every year to review their condition. Consequently, after 10 years of practice, an orthopaedic surgeon would need to see 1000 patients annually just to check that everything is still satisfactory. The logistics involved are complicated and the costs of implementing an adequate follow-up system are frequently prohibitive. This is why few centres in the world are able to collect and collate accurate data. None the less, if an orthopaedic unit is taking total hip replacement seriously, then some facility should rightly exist for ensuring that detailed follow-ups of all patients are maintained after their operations. Only then will problems be highlighted at an early stage.

There are different methods of assessing the performance of a total hip replacement. At the simplest level it is a matter of how a patient feels about the operation, which is, perhaps, the most accurate method of assessment. Hip replacements can also be scored, putting a figure to the functioning of the hip replacement. A number of different scoring systems exist around the world, but they do not cover every aspect of hip replacement. However, they do allow for generalizations about the performance of hip replacements to be made. One commonly used score is the Harris Hip Score, named after a surgeon in America. The higher the score, then the better the hip is performing. As years go by, so scores can sometimes decline, representing a gradual failure of the replacement.

However, whichever design of hip replacement has been used, it still takes time for problems to appear. It is unusual for a hip replacement to fail, say, within one year of surgery. Indeed, failure within five or six years is also unusual.

There may be a difference between the patient's perception of failure and what a surgeon sees as failure. Usually, the two are in broad agreement in that when the clinical signs and X-ray changes indicate that the hip is beginning to fail, then the patient is normally beginning to feel discomfort. However, this is not always the case. In a few patients, there is *silent failure*. The X-rays show changes that point to failure occurring, but the patient feels nothing. This is a difficult situation for the orthopaedic surgeon to handle. Should a revision operation be performed on the basis of an X-ray or should it wait until the patient feels pain? There is frequent debate in orthopaedic circles as to which approach is best.

Because total hip replacements do last for many years, despite progressive failure, orthopaedic surgeons frequently talk in terms of the *survivorship* of a prosthesis. This is an estimate of the percentage of components that are still functioning well a given number of years after their insertion. By using methods of *survivorship analysis*, it is possible to predict how a hip replacement is likely to fare without waiting for ten years or more. Despite this, most reputable orthopaedic journals will not publish results of new hip replacements until a minimum of five to six years' follow-up data is available.

Many factors determine the lifespan of a total hip replacement. The age of the patient is important. The younger the patient, the shorter a hip replacement is likely to last. An American study reported in 1983 looked at more than 100 patients under the age of 45 at the time of their hip replacements. An average of 4½ years after the procedure, only 76 per cent of the replacements were still satisfactory. For this reason, great care and caution is needed if total hip replacements are performed for such young patients.

Obesity may be another cause of premature failure. If a patient is obese, the replacement operation itself can take significantly longer to perform and it may be harder to insert the components. Some surgeons even refuse to operate on patients who are significantly overweight because of this. Others do not. Whatever decision is made, it is important that obese patients are warned that their weight may shorten the lifespan of the replacement. The chances of short-term complications may be much higher. This can be a difficult situation for the patient, as the pain of osteoarthritis limits mobility, this reduces the amount of exercise they can do, which, in turn, exacerbates their obesity.

Component design may also influence the lifespan of a hip

replacement. Many designs have appeared on the market, have been inserted into patients and yet no scientific studies have been done to support their use. On a worldwide basis, only the minority of available designs have known long-term results, yet it is the long-term predictability of a hip replacement that should determine its use, not the fact that it is theoretically a good idea. It is its performance in practice that is important, not the theory, though theory naturally plays its part.

The failure of hip replacements does appear to increase with time. Some studies suggest that the failure rate at 15 years is more than twice that at 10 years. Also, different parts of the total hip replacement behave in different ways. The femoral component usually lasts longer than does the acetabular component. Indeed, it is the problem of failure of the cemented acetabular component that has led orthopaedic surgeons to look at the use of cementless acetabular components. Long-term results of modern cementless acetabular components are not as yet available. However, short-term survivorship studies suggest that its success up to six and a half years later is equal to that of its cemented counterpart. Only time will tell whether it does better than the cemented design in the long term.

The cemented femoral component, however, does well — particularly if modern cementing techniques are used. At the time of writing, the author is unaware of any cementless femoral component with long-term results better than those of the best cemented designs.

Surgical technique plays a significant part in the longevity of a total hip replacement. Results for the same design of component, inserted in different orthopaedic centres, show failure rates that vary between 1 and 24 per cent, with some very old-fashioned designs having done well in the long-term — perhaps because of the expertise with which they were inserted.

Such variations in results between different centres have led some surgeons to call for the creation of specialist hip units, performing only joint replacements. Due to the numbers involved, however, it is unlikely that such units could be set up. Nevertheless, it is understandable that the more a surgeon performs a particular operation, the better their technique is likely to become. Proficient surgical technique is vital for long-lasting hip replacements.

You would not expect a revision hip replacement to last as long as a primary one and this is indeed the case, though some centres claim that the results of a first revision are as good as the results of a primary replacement. Certainly, the early results of revision surgery can be as good as the results of a primary procedure, but, overall, the failure rate of a revision replacement is higher. For revisions of revisions, the failure rate can be as high as 60 per cent. It is because of the poor results of revision operations that surgeons frequently attempt to delay the primary procedure for as long as possible because, once a primary hip replacement has been performed, there is no going back.

10

AFTER THE OPERATION

Surgery forms only part of what happens when a patient goes to hospital for a hip replacement. While in hospital, treatment is received from nursing staff, physiotherapists, occupational therapists, social workers and others. Even though most patients remain in hospital for approximately ten days after their operation, recovery is probably not complete in all respects until three months later. Only then is a patient likely to feel that all their physical and mental faculties are back to normal, even though they will be able to be up and about within 48 hours of the operation.

This chapter will cover what happens post-operatively in the three main phases of recovery:

1 in hospital
2 11 days to 6 weeks after the operation
3 six weeks to three months after the operation.

It is important to remember that treatment regimes vary from surgeon to surgeon and from one orthopaedic unit to another. There is no single, *correct* system for looking after a hip replacement patient, just as there is no single right way to drive a car. What follows is a reflection of my own practice and it is a very common way for patients to be looked after.

In Hospital

On returning to the ward the patient will have an intravenous drip in place and a number of drain tubes leading from the incision to bottles attached to the side of the bed. Drain tubes may not always be used, however.

It is usual for the patient to lie down on their back, often with some form of spacing pillow between the legs (the *abduction pillow* mentioned earlier). This keeps the hip stable until the patient is fully awake again. Nursing staff are also likely to continually remind the patient to lie on their back, as it is instinctive for many people to lie on their side while in bed.

The anaesthetist will have administered painkilling (*analgesic*) and antisickness (*anti-emetic*) medication before the patient is returned to the ward. Such treatment will continue while the patient requires it. In many hospitals, *patient-controlled analgesia* (PCA) is offered. With this, patients administer their own analgesics (under strict guidance from medical staff). Post-operative doses of antibiotics are also given at this stage to minimize the chances of infection. DVT stockings are put on the patient's legs by nursing staff (if they have been removed at the time of the operation) to help avoid DVTs (see pages 87 – 8) developing. These may be worn for up to six weeks after the operation, at which point the risk of a DVT developing is minimal.

Though the patient will have had nothing to eat for at least six hours prior to the operation, some sort of nourishment is given fairly soon afterwards. Initially, this is in the form of sips of liquid only, but light foods are normally given on the first day after the operation. By the second day, a normal diet is likely to be offered. The only exception is if there are any gastrointestinal problems, such as ileus (see page 86).

THE FIRST DAY AFTER THE OPERATION

Analgesics, anti-emetics and preventative treatment for DVTs continue. Light foods are introduced and some movement of the hip is attempted. Normally, a maximum of 45 degrees of movement is allowed at this stage. Some patients will find this difficult so early on, but it is important at this stage that medical staff teach the patient to be confident about their new hip. Also, becoming mobile as soon as possible reduces the chances of DVTs forming.

Blood tests are performed to assess the haemoglobin level. As a result of surgery, this can decline in a minority of cases, indicating that a blood transfusion may be needed. Meanwhile, paramedical staff are already beginning to make plans for when the patient returns home as a number of pieces of specialist equipment may be required.

THE SECOND DAY AFTER THE OPERATION

The same medication is given as on the first day, though the amount of anti-emetics and the strength of the analgesics administered are likely to be reduced. Drains are also likely to be removed, unless there is still a significant quantity of fluid leaking out of the incision.

At this stage, most patients will get out of bed for the first time, and then the hip joint will be allowed to move through approximately 70 degrees – sitting will not be permitted, though, except on a commode. For the first time, the patient will be shown how to use walking aids, most likely a walking frame.

By the second day, the result of the haemoglobin test will be known and action can be taken if the level is low. A low haemoglobin result does not always mean that a blood transfusion is necessary. For minor reductions in haemoglobin level, it is best to leave Nature to do her work. For moderate reductions, then a return of the haemoglobin to the normal level can be achieved by taking iron supplements. Only with severe reductions in haemoglobin is a blood transfusion required.

A hip X-ray may be taken, known as the *check X-ray*. It is mainly used as a record so that future X-rays can be checked against it to monitor whether or not any changes are occurring. Some hospitals choose not to have a patient move until the check X-ray has been done, though such a precaution is probably unnecessary. In certain countries, it is traditional to take an X-ray on the operating table, during the operation itself, to ensure that everything is as it should be before the patient recovers from the anaesthetic.

THE THIRD DAY AFTER THE OPERATION

The giving of analgesics, anti-emetics and preventative treatment for DVTs continue, though the DVT treatment is likely to be given by injection, while the analgesics and anti-emetics are likely to be taken orally. The intravenous drip will now be removed, unless a blood transfusion is needed. The patient will now be on a normal diet, be allowed to sit in a chair and to walk, with support, distances of up to 20 m (22 yds). Beyond regular checks on temperature and blood pressure, no special tests are required at this stage.

THE FOURTH DAY AFTER THE OPERATION

The giving of analgesics continues, as does preventative DVT treatment. The diet is normal, and the patient can get about with the aid of crutches rather than a frame. Beyond routine checks, no specific tests are required.

At about this time, though sometimes a little later, discussions will be held with the patient, or family and friends, as to what facilities are available at home. For example, is the toilet seat a low one? Are there only low chairs at home? Are there handles on the bath? Answers to all these kinds of questions are vital to ensuring that the patient recovers well from the operation. Many people find it difficult to recall exactly what is at home when asked, so it is helpful if patients know the answers to these questions *before* being admitted to hospital.

This work is largely the domain of the *occupational therapist*. It is their job to establish what equipment and specialist items may be required after the patient leaves hospital and to consider which services they may need. The patient may also be given a number of tips and shown some tricks to make washing and dressing, moving from place to place and so on easier. For those living alone, the therapist will also assess whether or not they will be able to manage in their kitchen as it is. To assess everything adequately, it is sometimes necessary for the occupational therapist to visit the patient's home.

THE FIFTH TO SEVENTH DAYS AFTER THE OPERATION

Preventative DVT treatment continues, with analgesics being administered only if required. A normal diet is offered and mobility gradually increases at this stage. Crutches are used in preference to a walking frame, but the patient is now becoming more responsible for their own daily exercises.

THE EIGHTH DAY AFTER THE OPERATION

Preventative DVT treatment continues. It is unlikely that anything other than mild analgesics will be required at this stage. Mobility continues to increase, with attention being paid to managing stairs on crutches. This can be quite an art, not everyone learning the technique first time.

Any specialist items of equipment identified by the patient and occupational therapist should now have been delivered (see Figure 10.1), either to the hospital or to the patient's home.

Final discharge details are organized, such as how the patient is to get home, who will do the cooking at home, shopping and so on.

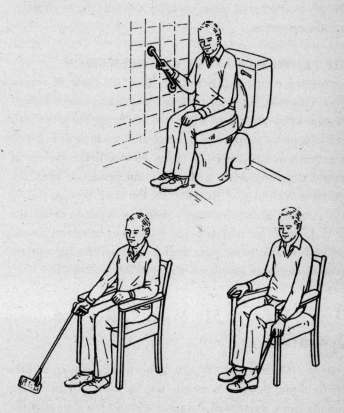

Figure 10.1 *Special aids and devices may be needed once at home.*

THE NINTH DAY AFTER THE OPERATION

Analgesics are only occasionally required at this stage, though preventative DVT treatment continues. A normal diet is offered and the patient can now get about independently and is able to negotiate stairs.

Letters are now being prepared for those who will be involved in the patient's care once they are at home.

Preparations are also made for the removal of the stitches or staples, which will occur on approximately the twelfth day after the operation.

THE TENTH DAY AFTER THE OPERATION

For most patients, this is the day they are likely to return home. However, there are obvious exceptions to the rule, and different units differ as to when they are happy for patients to be discharged – people stay in hospital for as little as five days to as much as two weeks or more. However, the process of gradually reintroducing a patient's independence after the operation is similar in all units. By the time they go home, most patients are independently mobile and able to undertake the majority of normal daily activities for themselves. Should they not be able to do this, then it is likely that appropriate home support will have been arranged by the hospital.

Eleven Days to Six Weeks after the Operation

Patients often expect to return to normality as soon as they return home, but this is usually not the case. For most, the pain of osteoarthritis will disappear within a few days after the operation, but some residual discomfort still remains. It is likely that the hip joint area will be slightly uncomfortable for at least six weeks afterwards. Swelling of the ankle or ankles can occur, as can occasional episodes of knee pain. All of this is normal and the patient should not be alarmed if they feel discomfort during this period. Some surgeons insist on the preventative DVT treatment being continued when the patient has returned home, which may take the form of a daily injection being given by a visiting nurse or the wearing of a supportive leg stocking. Other surgeons finish such treatment by the time of discharge.

This period is also a potentially dangerous time. The patient no longer has the guidance and assistance of nursing and paramedical staff. While in hospital, patients understand the importance of not flexing their hip joint too far. The chairs and beds there are suitably high, thereby minimizing the chance of the hip dislocating. Once home, however, there is no physiotherapist or nurse immediately on hand to correct the patient if this should be necessary. The patient's favourite chair, maybe one they have used for years, might be a low one and, obviously, they will want to use it. It is very difficult for a patient to avoid falling into their old habits. It is thus strongly recommended that hip replacement patients discipline themselves at this stage and take *no* risks until after their first out-patient consultation with their surgeon.

Six Weeks to Three Months after the Operation

At six weeks, most patients are seen by their surgeon. Stitches will have been removed and the patient should be independently mobile, using either a walking stick or crutch for support. The only exception will be if it has been necessary to limit the amount of weight borne by the new hip, say when bone grafting is performed during the operation or when certain cementless designs are used. Should this have been the case, the first out-patient appointment with the surgeon is likely to be the point when significant weight-bearing will be permitted, but, anyway, it is unusual for this to be limited for anything more than three months after the operation. However, for the majority of patients who have undergone a routine primary hip replacement, the six-week out-patient review is when life is allowed to return to almost total normality (for further details, see Chapter 13).

It should be remembered that energy levels are unlikely to be as before until about three months after the operation. The elderly, particularly, may feel sleepy and lethargic at this stage, but this is normal – due to the combination of having undergone a major operation, general anaesthetic and a period of time in hospital.

Taking Care of a Replacement Hip

Good though a hip replacement may be, there is one restriction that comes with it that is likely to remain for life – the need to avoid dislocating it.

The chances of this happening are always there, though they are greater shortly after the operation than they are several months later. However, it is wise for all patients to bear in mind that a significant risk of dislocation exists whenever the hip joint is flexed to an angle of 90 degrees or more. Restricting the range of movement of a hip joint is not a handicap and, indeed, the majority of patients cope with this well and do not notice any limitations. Nevertheless, the risk of dislocation should always be borne in mind and avoiding action taken accordingly.

There are certain occasions when dislocation is more likely to occur than at other times. Picking up items from the floor, for example, involves bending right down, which can cause dislocation. Putting on socks, stockings and shoes can also cause problems. Using sock and stocking aids, tights aids, long-handled shoe horns and easy reachers can help avoid stressing the joint too much.

For this reason, high chairs should be used wherever possible (the exact height required will depend on the patient's own height). The ideal chair will not flex the hip more than 90 degrees from the vertical. For the average person, the height of the seat should be at least 49 cm (19 in) from the floor to be safe. Chairs and beds with free-standing legs can be raised by simply using wooden blocks, but those with casters will need to be adapted in other ways. Toilet seats should also be higher than usual and a toilet surround frame is useful, too.

Getting in to and out of a bath must be done carefully after a hip replacement operation. Handles on the bath and adjacent walls, bath boards, bath seats and a non-slip mat in the bath itself are all very useful.

The occupational therapist is a mine of helpful information on how to do all sorts of things safely, and patients can do a lot to help themselves. Taking the following precautions, for life, will greatly reduce the chances of the replacement hip dislocating:

- do not cross your legs (knees or ankles)
- do not bend the hip beyond a right angle (90 degrees)
- do not sit on low stools, chairs or toilets
- do not sit on armless chairs as you need the arms to push on in order to stand
- only get out of a chair after having first moved to the edge of it, keep the leg of the operated on hip in front while getting up, and push on the arms of the chair to get out of it
- do not twist the hip inwards or outwards

- do not pick up objects from the floor without either using a special appliance or placing the leg of the operated on side straight behind you
- do not jump
- do not pivot on the leg of the operated on side
- do not stretch forwards from a sitting position
- avoid lifting heavy things
- do not put on excess weight.

11

PHYSIOTHERAPY

Physiotherapy plays a vital part in the convalescence of the hip replacement patient. Not only does it help in the expected physical ways, but it also gives immense psychological support. Hip replacement can be a frightening operation for patients, who may not be sure that everything is going to plan. The physiotherapist can help greatly in this respect, inspiring confidence and cooperation at a time when most patients feel fairly helpless.

As well as the work specifically aimed at helping the hip area to function normally again, physiotherapy also encourages better, deeper breathing and counteracts the sluggish blood flow that can occur when you spend time in hospital. These are important in order to prevent respiratory infections and DVTs occurring. It is for this reason that breathing and foot and ankle exercises are encouraged after the operation. Breathing exercises help the lungs push secretions away into the breathing tubes and then these secretions can be cleared away by coughing. If they stay in the lungs, infection can set in. Deep breathing and gentle coughing should therefore be encouraged, at least until the third day after the operation.

Foot and ankle exercises should be done regularly while the

patient is in hospital. Until someone is fully mobile again, the risk of DVTs forming continues to exist. The more active the foot and ankle are, the less likely it is that blood clots will form in the veins in the calf.

The physiotherapist will normally see the patient on the first day after the operation. The patient will then be encouraged to move the new hip gently, albeit with help. The gradual progression towards mobility that takes place over the next few days should occur under the strict eye of a physiotherapist. As the days go by, the patient will become more independently mobile and less reliant on the physiotherapist.

Exercises to do Following a Hip Replacement Operation

EXERCISES TO DO IN BED

These exercises are to do immediately after the operation and for at least six weeks afterwards. They are performed sitting in bed with the back supported by a back-rest inclined at approximately 45 degrees. Exercises 1 to 4 should be performed ten times every hour while you are awake. Exercises 5 to 7 should be repeated ten times each, four times a day.

1 With the legs straight, pull your foot up towards you until your toes are pointing to the ceiling. Then point your toes and feet down towards the end of the bed. Stretch your feet and toes each way as far as possible.
2 Circle both feet round in each direction.
3 Tighten the muscles in both your thighs, pushing your knees down firmly into the bed.
4 Squeeze your buttock muscles tightly together, then relax.
5 Bend your hip and knee gently upwards, then lower

slowly. Do not pull your leg up by hand. Do not bend the hip joint to more than a right angle. It may be necessary to use a sliding board to assist with this exercise (a sliding board is one on which the heel can slide, to avoid the friction that the heel would create sliding against a sheet).

6 Lay your legs straight out in front of you, then tighten the muscles and slide your leg towards the edge of the bed and back again (but do not move the leg across an imaginary line running down the centre of our body, do not *roll* your leg outwards and keep your toes pointed towards the ceiling throughout).

7 Place a rolled up towel under your knee. Straighten your leg, tensing the muscles so that your heel lifts up off the bed, keeping the back of your knee in contact with the towel at all times. Lower your heel slowly back to rest on the bed.

EXERCISES TO DO SITTING AND STANDING

These exercises should only be performed when you are able to sit or stand independently.

Sitting

1 Sitting on a high chair, slide your bottom to the front of the chair. Both feet should be firmly placed on the floor and take great care not to bend the hip through more than 90 degrees. Straighten your leg and tense your muscles to raise your foot off the floor. Keep your toes pointed up towards the ceiling and hold the position for five seconds. Then lower your leg carefully towards the floor.

2 Adopt the same position as in exercise 1 above. Lean back against the back of the chair and gently lift up your thigh, raising your foot from the floor and keeping your knee bent. Do not flex your hip through more than a right

angle. Then, lower your leg, putting your foot back on
the floor. Do not pull your leg up with your hands.

Standing

The following exercises are for the operated on leg only. You
should stand straight, though it may be necessary to hold on to
something to balance. The upper body should not be moved
and the moving foot should not touch the floor during these
exercises.

1 Keeping your leg straight, slowly swing your leg forwards
   and backwards, leaning ever so slightly to the opposite
   side so it can swing without touching the floor.
2 Swing your leg sideways away from the body and then
   back to the centre. Keep your kneecap facing forwards at
   all times and do not cross your legs.
3 Swing your leg gently round in a circle – front, side,
   behind and return.
4 Swing your leg forwards to an angle of 45 degrees from
   the vertical and hold that position for a count of five.
   Then lower your leg and swing it gently back as far as
   possible. Hold that position for a count of five and then
   lower.
5 Swing your leg out to the side to an angle of 45 degrees
   from the vertical and hold it there for a count of five.
   Then lower. Do not let your leg come further back in
   than the centre of your body and keep your upper body
   still.

These exercises, in the sitting *and* standing positions, should
be performed ten times each, four times a day. They should
continue to be done for at least six weeks after the operation.

Looking after the New Hip

To ensure that the new hip is moved safely, the patient will need to learn a number of techniques to complete otherwise familiar activities.

GETTING IN TO AND OUT OF BED

Always get in to and out of bed on the side of the operated on leg. The legs should be kept well apart and you should lean back as you move to avoid excessive bending of the hip.

When getting out of bed, it is best to perch on the side of the bed, keeping the operated on leg out in front until you have reached a standing position. To get in to bed, simply do the reverse of this.

GETTING IN TO AND OUT OF A CHAIR

Choose a chair that has a high seat, is firm and has arms. When you want to sit down, feel first for the arms of the chair, letting the operated on leg slide out in front as you do so. Sit on the front edge of the chair, then slide your bottom gently backwards into the chair.

Getting out of the chair simply involves reversing this procedure. The same technique should also be used when you need to go to the toilet.

WALKING

For at least six weeks after the operation, some form of support is required when you walk. Occasionally, a surgeon will request that the patient always use some form of support when walking.

When using a frame or a pair of crutches or walking sticks and you want to walk forwards, do the following.

- First, place your frame or walking aid securely ahead of you, then move your operated on leg, then your unoperated on leg.
- If you want to turn in a confined space, turn towards your *unoperated* on side to prevent twisting your new hip.

STAIRS

These are best climbed using crutches, rather than a walking frame. Only one step should be negotiated at a time. To go upstairs, do the following.

- Place your crutches securely each side of you, then move the unoperated on leg on to the step, then the operated on leg, then follow with the crutches.

To go downstairs, the sequence is as follows.

- Move the crutches downwards ahead of you and make sure they are stable. Follow with the operated on leg, then the unoperated on leg.

GETTING IN TO AND OUT OF A CAR

To get in to a car, first, push the seat back as far as possible and slightly recline it. Lower yourself slowly down to the edge of the seat, with your back towards the opposite door. Push yourself backwards towards the opposite door in order to allow you to keep your operated on leg as straight as possible as you slide round into the seat. Keep leaning backwards as you do so, keeping the leg straight and turning carefully as you lower your leg and place your foot in the footwell.

To get out of the car, reverse this procedure, though make sure you hold your operated on leg out in front of you before you stand up.

12

NURSING CARE

Nurses are the backbone of any healthcare team and, arguably, the care they give is the most important aspect of a patient's stay in hospital. Without it, a carefully planned and executed operation can come to nought.

A patient undergoing a hip replacement operation will meet with nurses in four different areas of the healthcare system:

- out-patients
- ward
- operating theatre
- community.

In whichever area they work, all nurses undergo a similar basic training.

Out-patient Nurses

When a patient first meets their orthopaedic surgeon, the setting is normally a busy out-patient clinic. This clinic is largely run and controlled by nursing staff. Nurses are generally responsible for preparing the patient prior to seeing the specialist and will often be in attendance throughout the consultation.

The first meeting with a specialist can be a confusing occasion and the out-patient nurse is therefore very involved in answering the various questions patients have.

Ward Nurses

On admission to the ward, the patient can be faced by a confusing array of nurses, all in differently coloured uniforms and with different titles. There is a distinct pecking order within the nursing hierarchy. Most wards, or ward areas, are run by a nursing sister. The sister may be answerable to a manager above them, but beneath them are varying numbers of qualified nurses. The qualified nurses have different names in different countries, but in the United Kingdom are normally referred to as staff nurses. Beneath the staff nurses will be a variable number of student nurses, auxiliary nurses, enrolled nurses and hospital volunteers.

There are different nursing systems in different countries and different hospitals. One system is the *primary* nursing system. Here, a nurse specializes in a given area (in this case orthopaedic surgery) and is entirely responsible for the nursing care of certain selected patients during the working day.

In other systems, a patient will be cared for by a number of different nurses, though there is now a tendency within healthcare systems to ensure that patients are looked after by a particular, named nurse. That nurse is responsible for coordinating the patient's entire stay in hospital – from nursing care, to liaising with relatives, from the time they come on to the ward until they go home.

Being in hospital can be a time when patients feel very

helpless, which is a shock when you are normally used to being in control of your own destiny. The nurse will smooth the way for the hip replacement patient while they are in hospital, making things much easier to cope with.

In recent times, the nursing profession has assumed much greater responsibility for the care of patients than was the case a decade ago. Decisions concerning medication are now frequently made autonomously by nursing staff (drugs are changed, intravenous drips resited and so on) as they are very experienced. In previous times, all such tasks were considered suitable only to be performed by doctors.

The ward nurse, as well as fulfilling her role of general carer, may also act as an interim physiotherapist. Though a physiotherapist is likely to visit the hip replacement patient most days before and after surgery, the nurse will see the patient more frequently, so it will be the nurse who encourages the patient to do the exercises in bed. Also, it will be the nurse who will help the patient to walk once out of bed.

Prior to the operation, it is the ward nurse's responsibility to ensure that all the required documentation is in order. This is vital for hip replacement patients, as it must be clearly established which side is to be operated on. This may seem obvious, but when someone comes to hospital for a hip replacement, they need to visit a number of different hospital areas. On entering each area, the care of the patient is transferred to another member of staff. If things are unclear, you have problems, so a large arrow is often drawn on the person's affected limb for all to see.

Consent is also required for the operation. Although this part of the form-filling process is often performed by junior medical staff, none the less, the nurse needs to ensure that consent has been obtained before the patient leaves the ward for operating theatre. It will also be her job to ensure that the patient's skin is prepared for surgery and that shaving, if required, is also undertaken.

After the hip replacement operation, a patient will spend quite some time in bed. Though the patient will begin to walk on the second day after the operation, this is only done for a little while – the rest of the time being spent either in bed or sitting in a chair. This can lead to pressure sores (see page 91), so nursing staff do as much as possible to avoid these forming, ensuring that patients change position regularly, to relieve pressure on at-risk areas. If a pressure sore does develop despite their efforts, this can delay a patient's return home until it clears up, which can take several weeks. This is why, as we saw earlier, nursing staff may assess patients' chances of developing the problem before they have their operations. If the patient is shown to be significantly at risk, then the nurses take extra care with that patient and a special kind of mattress may be supplied for the bed to help avoid one forming. Such a patient can also expect to be handled extra carefully for the first two to three days after the operation. Two, or even three, nurses will lift the patient clear of the bed for several minutes on a regular basis to alleviate pressure on the more sensitive areas. In some orthopaedic units, patients may be rolled onto their sides to achieve the same effect, though this must naturally be done in a strictly controlled way after a hip replacement operation.

A ward nurse may also need to measure the patient for DVT stockings prior to the operation. Stockings come in various sizes and must be neither too tight nor too loose if they are to prevent DVTs forming.

Once the patient has been greeted, assessed and prepared by the nurse, it is then time for them to put on an operating theatre gown. Then the pre-medication prescribed by the anaesthetist is given. The patient is then wheeled to the operating theatre, normally accompanied by the ward nurse, who may remain with the patient until the anaesthetic has been given.

After the operation, the ward nurse will monitor the patient's blood pressure, temperature and pulse at least every half hour for the first two hours after the patient has returned to the ward. For three to four days thereafter, such measurements will be taken every four hours. It is all the measurements taken together that make assessment easier. Just after the operation, for example, a patient will frequently develop a small rise in temperature. If this is a simple spike on the temperature chart, then there is no need for concern. However, if the temperature stays at a higher than normal level, then this can sometimes indicate that there is a need for further investigation. Thus it is important that the nurses measure and chart vital signs carefully.

Also, the incision will be checked to ensure that there is not too much fluid seeping from it and the general colour of the limbs will be observed to ensure that the circulation is good.

As we have seen, the administration of the medication prescribed for the patients is also the responsibility of the ward nurse. Generally, the nurse will not prescribe the drugs, though she will certainly administer them. It is the nurse's job, with colleagues, to check and double-check that the medicines and dosages are correct.

Just after the operation, a patient will have a fine intravenous tube in place. Occasionally, this may be used to transfuse blood, but it is more usual to have an infusion of a clear fluid such as saline. The nurse ensures that the intravenous drip is running smoothly and that the bags of sterile fluid are changed at the appropriate times.

The abduction pillow that has been placed between the legs after the operation sometimes shifts its position. The nurse will check it frequently and move it as necessary to ensure that the patient's legs are held in a safe position for the new hip for the first few days after the operation.

By approximately the third day after the operation, the ward nurse will probably reduce the size of the patient's dressing. After the new hip has been inserted, the surgeon will cover the incision with a large dressing so that gentle pressure is applied to the skin and deeper tissues in order to minimize bleeding. There is usually no longer a need for such a large dressing more than two days after the operation. By the third day, it is therefore customary to replace it with a smaller one. Attention to how the site of the incision is healing continues throughout the patient's stay in hospital, though the number of changes of dressings lessens as it heals. It is possible that the incision will ooze for several days after the operation, but this should not cause concern, though more frequent changing of the dressings may be needed.

Life on a ward can appear very hectic to a patient. Indeed, orthopaedic wards can be busy, with a continual flow of patients on to and off the ward. A shift system is normally worked by nursing staff. Such shifts can sometimes be quite long, but if a patient's normal nurse disappears, this probably means that their shift has come to an end. It is unlikely to mean that the nurse is being intentionally neglectful.

Theatre Nurses

Theatre nursing staff form an integral part of the operating team. The nurse who hands the surgeon instruments is the theatre sister, or *scrub nurse*. She will have seen large numbers of total hip replacement operations, may well have been first assistant at many of them and will be familiar with the techniques used by the surgeon concerned. If there is any suggestion that the scrub nurse does not have sufficient experience, then a more experienced nurse will work alongside them.

Because the scrub nurse has scrubbed up and so is clean and sterile, they are unable to leave the patient's side. If any instruments or sutures need to be fetched during the operation, this is done by a *circulating nurse*. The circulating nurse has not scrubbed up and so can fetch instruments that may be needed during the operation that are not immediately to hand. The technique for passing an instrument from the unsterile circulating nurse to the sterile scrub nurse, while still maintaining the sterility of the instrument, is one that takes time to learn, but learning it is a vital part of the operation as a whole. However careful the surgeon may be in carrying out the operation, unsterile behaviour by any one of the nurses can result in infection being transmitted to the patient. Once an infection occurs, it is unlikely that the source of that infection will be able to be identified. Nurses in the operating theatre thus take their job of keeping everything and, in the case of the scrub nurse, themselves sterile very seriously.

Once the operation is over, the patient is transferred to the recovery ward. In the recovery ward will be a *recovery nurse*. The recovery nurse looks after the patient immediately after their operation until they are transferred back to the ward nurse.

Community Nurses

Once a patient has fully recovered from their operation, they will be discharged from hospital and return home, whether that be their own home, a convalescence centre or relatives and friends. Wherever they go, they often require some kind of nursing care. This is less intensive care than is received on the ward, obviously, but may involve the changing of dressings, removal of sutures or simply the giving of advice. All this will be done by the *community nurse*, who will frequently be based at a doctors' practice.

13

WHEN CAN I . . . ?

Hip replacement operations are performed to give patients a better quality of life. It is not surprising, therefore, that most are keen and eager to return to normality as soon as possible after their operations. At the same time, surgeons are keen to prevent their patients from doing too much at too early a stage. It is important to allow healing to be as complete as possible.

The possibility of dislocation is always a worry, however long ago the patient had their operation. Any activity that flex-es the hip to more than 90 degrees will put the joint at risk. Think of a hip replacement as if it were a new car — the more you use it, the more you abuse it, the sooner it will fail.

In the out-patient review clinics I run for my patients, I am frequently asked when it is appropriate for certain specific activities to be undertaken or resumed. There are no hard and fast rules, and common sense has much to do with the advice given at this stage. What follow are examples of many typical questions that are asked by patients after their operations. The answers given to them are the ones I would give and reflect my own practice — they are not necessarily answers others would give or the practice of others. The policies of different orthopaedic surgeons are as diverse as the number of hip replacement designs on the market today. So, before you take any risks at all, *ask your surgeon!*

When can I sleep on my side?

Six weeks after the operation. You are stopped from sleeping on your side for this time as most people curl up into a ball when they are asleep. This puts the hip at risk of dislocation and this risk is greatest when the hip operated on is upper-most.

When can I stop wearing my DVT stockings?

Six weeks after surgery. The risk of DVTs forming continues after you have been discharged from hospital, but six weeks after the operation, the risk is then tiny and so it should be safe to stop wearing them at that point.

When can I start having sex again?

What's keeping you?! However, take care for the first six weeks after the operation and don't be *too* acrobatic! Also, it is best if you are on the bottom, with your partner on top. Do not bend the hip operated on too far, though it is unlikely that you will dislocate it if your legs are apart.

When can I stop using a raised toilet seat?

Three months after the operation. It is necessary to use it up until then in order to avoid the risk of dislocating the new hip by bending it too much. Fortunately, hips rarely dislocate when the legs are kept apart. However, if you have only the very low, modern toilets, it may be worth considering installing higher ones.

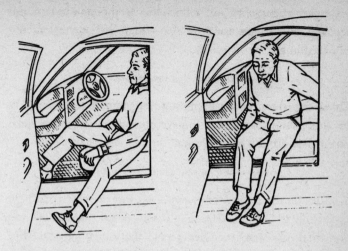

Figure 13.1 *Getting in to and out of a car needs to be done with care and following the steps practised with the physiotherapist.*

When can I drive my car?

Six weeks after the operation. However, get in and out of the car carefully (see Figure 13.1). Push your seat as far back as it will go and recline the backrest a few degrees. Keep your legs slightly apart when driving.

When can I sit on a low chair?

I would rather you *never* sat on a low chair after a hip operation. However, if there is no alternative, lean slightly backwards when you are seated and keep your legs apart.

When can I walk without my walking stick?

Six weeks after the operation, though with some cementless hips you may need to keep using one for three months. I would always keep a walking stick handy in future, though, as you never know when you will need it. Remember to hold the walking stick in the hand on the *opposite* side to that of the replaced hip.

When can I go swimming?

Three months after the operation. It is best if you use back-stroke or crawl, as neither require much hip movement. Take care if you use the breaststroke.

Can I ride a bicycle or an exercise bike?

Yes, three months after the operation. Put the seat up as high as possible to limit the degree of flexing of the hip needed, and don't fall off! Many surgeons forbid the use of bicycles after hip replacement, but I work in Cambridge, the home of the British bicycle, where bicycles are a way of life and I could not ban their use if I tried!

Can I ride a motorbike?

Yes, if you must. One of my patients did complete a circuit of the Isle of Man TT, but I would not *recommend* doing this.

Can I put on my own shoes, socks and stockings?

Yes, but three months after the operation. The hip joint needs to be flexed to an extreme angle to do these things and so the risk of dislocating it while doing them will always exist. It is best to use the opposite hand to the operated on leg when putting on socks and shoes. A long-handled shoe horn would be useful.

Can I cut my toenails?

The same problem exists here as in the previous question. You may have difficulty reaching down that far without putting your hip at risk of dislocating.

Can I kneel to say prayers?

Yes, six weeks after the operation. When most people pray, the hip joint is kept almost straight, even though the knees are bent. I haven't had any of my patients dislocate a hip in church as yet!

Can I do the gardening?

Yes, from six weeks after the operation onwards. However, remember to keep your hip straight. Using a kneeling stool would be a good idea.

My hip replacement aches from time to time. Does this mean it is going wrong?

Sometimes yes, but more usually no. It is normal to feel slight discomfort in your hip, buttock or thigh at times after the operation. This is particularly so when you have overused the joint. It highlights the fact that the word *replacement* is probably the wrong one; it is more accurate to say that you have an *artificial* hip, with its own different kinds of strengths and weaknesses.

Can I go on a walking holiday?

Yes, of course. But wait until three months after the operation and take a walking stick with you. Take care on rough, irregular ground and only carry a light rucksack.

Another specialist needs to operate on me. Is it safe?

Yes, provided your surgeon knows you have had a hip replacement. When you are under anaesthetic it is possible for your hip to dislocate unless special precautions are taken, so all concerned need to know about it even if the operation involves a totally separate part of the body. You may also need to take antibiotics to avoid any risk of infection.

This need for care can also apply to more minor procedures, such as having a tooth out, so I would recommend you discuss this with your surgeon or dentist.

Is it safe to have a baby?

Usually yes, though I would wait until at least six months after the operation. The womb is on the inside of the pelvis and the hip joint is on the outside of it so one should not interfere with the other. However, the delivery can cause problems if you forget to maintain your hips in the correct position in the heat of the moment. Discuss this with your obstetrician, who may wish to seek orthopaedic advice.

Can I fly or travel by bus and coach?

Yes, six weeks after the operation. However, I would try and ensure that you have lots of leg room so that you do not put the hip at risk of flexing more than 90 degrees.

Will I set off the security alarms at airports?

Not as far as I am aware. However, I did have one patient who had both hip joints replaced and one knee joint replaced who *did* set off an alarm at an international airport, so I imagine it depends on how much metal is inside you.

When can I have a bath?

Six weeks after the operation. I would prefer you to take showers instead until then.

Can I carry bags of shopping?

Of course, but it would be best to wait until six weeks after the operation before doing so.

When can I cross my legs again?

Never. If you cross your legs, you put yourself at risk of dislocation.

Can I return to sports?

It depends *which* sports you want to do! I would prefer it if you kept to the gentler sports such as golf, bowls or not too frantic tennis. I would certainly avoid contact sports. However, the following is a list of sports my patients have undertaken after their hip replacement operations. I would not recommend any of them as being suitable, exactly, but here goes anyway:

- cricket
- salmon fishing
- jogging
- marathon running
- weight-lifting
- deep-sea fishing
- scuba diving
- skiing
- parachuting
- bunjee jumping (astonishingly, this patient did not dislocate their hip!)

14

THE FUTURE

Some Thoughts

It is impossible to predict what will happen in the future. However, what is undoubtedly true is that the wheel has turned full circle in orthopaedic surgery. In the early days of hip replacements, metal-to-metal joints were considered appropriate. Then they went out of favour and now they are back in favour again. Surface arthroplasty – exemplified by the Smith-Petersen cup, in vogue in the 1940s – is also again being performed. The lay person would be forgiven for thinking that orthopaedic surgeons are not very good at making up their minds!

What is probably true is that our descendants will look back on modern-day joint replacement and regard it as a primitive art. However advanced we may think we are now, to them we will appear simplistic. Current research into joint replacement is aimed at reducing the risk of failure due to the causes mentioned in Chapter 5. The production of wear debris, for example, as we have seen causes significant loosening. Efforts are thus being made to improve materials, so that the production of wear debris is reduced.

Orthopaedic surgery went through a phase of favouring cemented hip replacement designs in the 1960s and 1970s and then passed through a phase of preferring cementless ones. Cemented ones are now the most popular as further research into cementing techniques and new cements has improved them. Efforts are being made to develop cements that behave in the same way as bone. Meanwhile, for those who believe in the future of a cementless hip system, research continues into developing a long-lasting cementless design. Hydroxyapatite coating, only recently more readily available, is holding its own in this respect. Whether it can compete with the *long-term* results of the established cemented designs is impossible to say at this stage.

Components that require only limited removal of bone during a hip operation are also being studied. Some would consider that the only parts of the hip joint that really need to be removed are the femoral head and acetabulum, that reaming out the upper femoral canal is not necessary. Thus, cup arthroplasty has returned, too.

Revision surgery is increasing in frequency and complexity. The future will undoubtedly see the development of improved revision techniques and improved instrumentation to go with them. For example, devices to ensure the rapid, safe removal of cement from the femoral canal and acetabulum will probably appear in the next ten years. Safer revision surgery will mean better long-term results for revision replacements.

However, perhaps the most significant likely development is a better appreciation by surgeons and manufacturers of the need for good data to support the use of a particular replacement hip design. The present lack of legislation on designs must surely be coming to a close. It is likely that more stringent regulations will be created to ensure that safety standards are met. Then designs will only be allowed to be used if specific follow-up results are available for them. Why, for example, if a well-cemented femoral component can be shown to last ten years, should any other component be permitted to be used at all? Manufacturers will then be under greater pressure to *prove* the merits of their designs.

As it becomes apparent that the results of hip replacement operations vary between different units, it is more likely that specialist hip replacement centres will appear. This would have significant financial implications for any healthcare system, but it is arguably the best way to ensure reliability of performance in the long term.

My final thought is that, one day, hip replacements may not be needed. Further research into osteoarthritis may reveal that it is caused by something that can be treated medically and, in time, avoided altogether. Strangely enough, for a surgeon, I hope so.

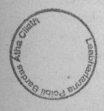

GLOSSARY

Abduction pillow
A flat, triangular cushion placed between the patient's legs after a hip replacement operation that ensures that the new joint is kept in a stable position until the patient regains independent control of their movements.

Acetabulum
Anatomical word for the socket of the hip joint.

Anteversion
Slightly forwards angle of the femoral neck at the upper end of the *femur*. The opposite of *retroversion*.

Arthrodesis
Surgical fusion of a joint.

Arthroplasty
Another word for joint replacement.

Arthroscopy
When a minute viewing telescope is used to inspect the inside of a joint.

Articular cartilage
The smooth, gristle covering of a bone that forms part of a joint.

Aseptic loosening
> Uninfected loosening of a joint replacement, usually caused by wear debris being produced in the socket.

Bearing surface
> The joint formed by the artificial ball and socket.

Bipolar replacement
> An all-in-one hip replacement, where the acetabular component is attached to the femoral ball in the factory. The acetabular component is not cemented into the patient's bone.

Bone banks
> Ultra-cold deep freezers where bone is stored until it is needed for grafting.

Bone stock
> The quality and consistency of bone. *Aseptic loosening* leads to reduced bone stock and corresponding bone weakness.

Cement mantle
> The layer of cement between the components of the replacement hip and the bone.

Check X-ray
> The X-ray taken after the new joint has been inserted to check that all is well.

Contracture
> A deformity of a joint, due to contraction of the soft tissues that surround it.

Cortex
> The hard outer shell of a bone.

Cortical perforation
> An accidental perforation of the cortex of a bone that can occur during surgery.

Custom components
> Tailor-made joint replacements.

Diathermy

An electrical device used to coagulate the blood during an operation.

Drain

Small tube left in the incision for a short while after the operation in order to allow surplus blood to drain away from the wound rather than collect within it.

Draping

The process of laying sterile towels over the patient in theatre, screening off unsterile areas from the sterile ones.

Femur

The thigh bone.

Fracture

A broken bone.

Fretting

The rubbing that takes place where two pieces of metal connect. An example of where this can happen would be the area between a modular metal ball and the spigot to which it is attached on the replacement femoral neck.

Haematoma

A collection of blood beneath the skin. It can pose a risk of infection.

Hemiarthroplasty

Replacement of only one side of a joint, for example of just the femoral component. Frequently performed when a patient has fractured their hip.

Hybrid total hip replacement

Combination of a cemented femoral component and a cementless acetabular component.

Hypertension

High blood pressure.

Hypotension

Low blood pressure.

Hypotensive anaesthesia
An anaesthetic technique whereby the patient's blood pressure is artificially lowered to reduce bleeding during the operation.

Hypothermia
Very low body temperature.

Induction
The act of administering anaesthetic to a patient.

Keyholes
Surgical pits created in the acetabular bone during a hip replacement operation that enable the cement to get a good hold on the bone.

Medulla
The soft, spongy, central portion of a bone.

Modularity
A component that can be assembled piece by piece during the operation, thereby enabling the surgeon to make individual adjustments to suit a particular patient.

Osteolysis
Destruction of bone, usually as a result of wear debris being created.

Osteophytes
Bony lips found at the margins of osteoarthritic joints.

Osteotomy
Surgical term meaning 'division of bone'.

PMMA
Abbreviation of *polymethylmethacrylate*.

Polymethylmethacrylate
Chemical used to make bone cement.

Porous coating
Tiny metal beads attached to the outer surface of a component to encourage integration by the surrounding bone. Used in cementless designs.

Pre-medication

Drug given immediately before the operation to make the patient drowsy and relaxed.

Primary replacement

The first hip replacement. After the primary replacement fails, *revision* operations are then performed.

Prosthesis

Another word for one of the components of a replacement hip joint.

Reaming

The surgical removal of bone to make a cavity in which the femoral or acetabular components can be inserted.

Retroversion

The slightly backwards angle of the femoral neck at the upper end of the *femur*. The opposite of *anteversion*.

Revision replacement

Any subsequent replacement on a hip joint done after the primary replacement has failed.

Salvage procedures

Last-ditch operations performed in an attempt to rescue a failing joint replacement.

Scrubbing-up

The cleaning of the hands and forearms carried out by the surgical team to render the skin as sterile as possible.

Sliding board

Smooth, friction-free board that is placed on a patient's bed to allow them to do their exercises after the operation. Otherwise, the sheets prevent the heel from sliding freely and the friction can be painful.

Synovium

The inner lining of a joint, responsible for the production and absorption of *synovial fluid*, which enables the joint to move freely.

Urinary retention
   Inability to pass urine due to its being retained in the bladder.

INDEX

Hip Replacement